Virtual Clinical Excursions—Medical Surgical

for

Ignatavicius and Workman:
Medical-Surgical Nursing:
Critical Thinking for Collaborative Care, 5th Edition

prepared by

Dorothy Mathers, RN, MSN
Associate Professor, Nursing
Pennsylvania College of Technology
Williamsport, Pennsylvania

software developed by

Wolfsong Informatics, LLC
Tucson, Arizona

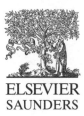

ELSEVIER
SAUNDERS

ELSEVIER
SAUNDERS

The Curtis Center
Independence Square West
Philadelphia, Pennsylvania 19106-3399

Notice

Nursing is an ever-changing field. Standard safety precautions must be followed, but as new research and
clinical experience broaden our knowledge, changes in treatment and drug therapy may become necessary
or appropriate. Readers are advised to check the most current product information provided by the manu-
facturer of each drug to be administered to verify the recommended dose, the method and duration of
administration, and contraindications. It is the responsibility of the licensed prescriber, relying on experience and knowledge of the patient, to determine dosages and the best treatment for each individual patient.
Neither the publisher nor the author assumes any liability for any injury and/or damage to persons or prop-
erty arising from this publication.

ISBN-13 978-1-4160-0103-4

ISBN-10 1-4160-0103-4

Senior Editor, Nursing: *Tom Wilhelm*
Managing Editor: *Jeff Downing*
Associate Developmental Editor: *Jennifer Anderson*
Project Manager: *Joy Moore*

Printed in the United States of America

Last digit is the print number: 9 8 7 6 5 4

Workbook
prepared by

Dorothy Mathers, RN, MSN
Associate Professor, Nursing
Pennsylvania College of Technology
Williamsport, Pennsylvania

Textbook

Donna D. Ignatavicius, MS, RNC, Cm
President, DI Associates, Inc.
Hughesville, Maryland
Former Professor
Charles County Community College
La Platta, Maryland

M. Linda Workman, PhD, RN, FAAN
Gertrude Perkins Oliva Professor of Oncology
Frances Payne Bolton School of Nursing
Case Western Reserve University
Cleveland, Ohio

Reviewer

Gina Long, RN, DNSc
Assistant Professor, Department of Nursing
College of Health Professions
Northern Arizona University
Flagstaff, Arizona

Contents

Table of Contents
Ignatavicius and Workman:
Medical-Surgical Nursing:
Critical Thinking for Collaborative Care, 5th Edition

Getting Started

GETTING SET UP

■ MINIMUM SYSTEM REQUIREMENTS

WINDOWS™

Windows Vista®, XP, 2000 (Recommend Windows XP/2000)
Pentium® III processor (or equivalent) @ 600 MHz (Recommend 800 MHz or better)
256 MB of RAM (Recommend 1 GB or more for Windows Vista®)
800 x 600 screen size (Recommend 1024 x 768)
Thousands of colors
12x CD-ROM drive
Soundblaster 16 soundcard compatibility
Stereo speakers or headphones

Note: Virtual Clinical Excursions—Medical-Surgical for Windows will require a minimal
amount of disk space to install icons and required dll files for Windows 98/ME. Windows Vista
and XP require administrator privileges for installation.

MACINTOSH®

MAC OS X (10.2 or higher)
Apple Power PC G3 @ 500 MHz or better
128 MB of RAM (Recommend 256 MB or more)
800 x 600 screen size (Recommend 1024 x 768)
Thousands of colors
12x CD-ROM drive
Stereo speakers or headphones

■ INSTALLATION INSTRUCTIONS

WINDOWS™

1. Insert the *Virtual Clinical Excursions—Medical-Surgical* CD-ROM.
2. The setup screen should appear automatically if the current product is not already installed. Windows Vista users may be asked to authorize additional security prompts.
3. Follow the onscreen instructions during the setup process.

   If the setup screen does *not* appear automatically (and *Virtual Clinical Excursions—Medical-Surgical* has not been installed already):
   a. Click the **My Computer** icon on your desktop or in your Start menu.
   b. Double-click on your CD-ROM drive.
   c. If installation does not start at this point:
      (1) Click the **Start** icon on the taskbar and select the **Run** option.
      (2) Type d:\setup.exe (where "d:\" is your CD-ROM drive) and press **OK**.
      (3) Follow the onscreen instructions for installation.

MACINTOSH®

1. Insert the *Virtual Clinical Excursions—Medical-Surgical* CD in the CD-ROM drive. The disk icon will appear on your desktop.

2. Double-click on the disk icon.

3. Double-click on the MEDICAL-SURGICAL_MAC run file.

Note: Virtual Clinical Excursions—Medical-Surgical for Macintosh does not have an installation setup and can only be run directly from the CD.

■ HOW TO USE VIRTUAL CLINICAL EXCURSIONS—MEDICAL-SURGICAL

WINDOWS™

1. Double-click on the *Virtual Clinical Excursions—Medical-Surgical* icon located on your desktop.
2. Or navigate to the program via the Windows Start menu.

Note: Windows 98/ME will require you to restart your computer before running the *Virtual Clinical Excursions—Medical-Surgical* program. Windows Vista computers require you to right-click on the desktop short-cut, choose Properties and in the Compatability Mode check the box for "Run as Administrator." Below is a screen capture to show what this looks like.

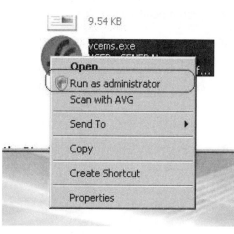

MACINTOSH®

1. Insert the *Virtual Clinical Excursions—Medical-Surgical* CD in the CD-ROM drive. The disk icon will appear on your desktop.

2. Double-click on the disk icon.

3. Double-click on the VCEMS_MAC run file.

Note: Virtual Clinical Excursions—Medical-Surgical for Macintosh does not have an installation setup and can only be run directly from the CD.

■ SCREEN SETTINGS

For best results, your computer monitor resolution should be set at a minimum of 800 x 600. The number of colors displayed should be set to "thousands or higher" (High Color or 16 bit) or "millions of colors" (True Color or 24 bit).

Windows™

1. From the **Start** menu, select **Control Panel** (on some systems, you will first go to **Settings**, then to **Control Panel**).
2. Double-click on the **Display** icon.
3. Click on the **Settings** tab.
4. Under **Screen resolution** use the slider bar to select **800 by 600 pixels**.
5. Access the **Colors** drop-down menu by clicking on the down arrow.
6. Select **High Color (16 bit)** or **True Color (24 bit)**.
7. Click on **OK**.
8. You may be asked to verify the setting changes. Click **Yes**.
9. You may be asked to restart your computer to accept the changes. Click **Yes**.

Macintosh®

1. Select the **Monitors** control panel.
2. Select **800 x 600** (or similar) from the **Resolution** area.
3. Select **Thousands** or **Millions** from the **Color Depth** area.

■ WEB BROWSERS

Supported web browsers include Microsoft Internet Explorer (IE) version 6.0 or higher, Netscape version 7.1 or higher, and Mozilla Firefox version 1.4 or higher.

If you use America Online (AOL) for web access, you will need AOL version 4.0 or higher and one of the browsers listed above. Do not use earlier versions of AOL with earlier versions of IE, because you will have difficulty accessing many features.

For best results with AOL:
- Connect to the Internet using AOL version 4.0 or higher.
- Open a private chat within AOL (this allows the AOL client to remain open, without asking whether you wish to disconnect while minimized).
- Minimize AOL.
- Launch a recommended browser.

■ TECHNICAL SUPPORT

Technical support for this product is available between 7:30 a.m. and 7 p.m. (CST), Monday through Friday. Before calling, be sure that your computer meets the minimum system requirements to run this software. Inside the United States and Canada, call 1-800-692-9010. Outside North America, call 314-872-8370. You may also fax your questions to 314-523-4932 or contact Technical Support through e-mail: technical.support@elsevier.com.

Trademarks: Windows, Macintosh, Pentium, and America Online are registered trademarks.

Copyright © 2005 by Elsevier, Inc.

All rights reserved. No part of this product may be reproduced or transmitted in any form or by any means, electronic or mechanical, including input or storage in any information system, without written permission from the publisher.

ACCESSING *Virtual Clinical Excursions—Medical-Surgical* FROM EVOLVE

The product you have purchased is part of the Evolve family of online courses and learning resources. Please read the following information thoroughly to get started.

To access your instructor's course on Evolve:

Your instructor will provide you with the username and password needed to access this specific course on the Evolve Learning System. Once you have received this information, please follow these instructions:

1. Go to the Evolve student page (http://evolve.elsevier.com/student)

2. Enter your username and password in the **Login to My Evolve** area and click the **Login** button.

3. You will be taken to your personalized **My Evolve** page, where the course will be listed in the **My Courses** module.

TECHNICAL REQUIREMENTS

To use an Evolve course, you will need access to a computer that is connected to the Internet and equipped with web browser software that supports frames. For optimal performance, it is recommended that you have speakers and use a high-speed Internet connection. However, slower dial-up modems (56 K minimum) are acceptable.

Whichever browser you use, the browser preferences must be set to enable cookies and JavaScript and the cache must be set to reload every time.

Enable Cookies

Browser	Steps
Internet Explorer (IE) 6.0 or higher	1. Select **Tools → Internet Options**. 2. Select **Privacy** tab. 3. Use the slider (slide down) to **Accept All Cookies**. 4. Click **OK**. -OR- 3. Click the **Advanced** button. 4. Click the check box next to **Override Automatic Cookie Handling**. 5. Click the **Accept** radio buttons under **First-party Cookies** and **Third-party Cookies**. 6. Click **OK**.
Netscape 7.1 or higher	1. Select **Edit → Preferences**. 2. Select **Privacy & Security**. 3. Select **Cookies**. 4. Select **Enable All Cookies**.
Mozilla Firefox 1.4 or higher	1. Select **Tools → Options**. 2. Select the **Privacy** icon. 3. Click to expand Cookies. 4. Select **Allow sites to set cookies**. 5. Click **OK**.

Enable JavaScript

Browser	Steps
Internet Explorer (IE) 6.0 or higher	1. Select **Tools → Internet Options**. 2. Select **Security** tab. 3. Under **Security level for this zone** set to **Medium** or lower.
Netscape 7.1 or higher	1. Select **Edit → Preferences**. 2. Select **Advanced**. 3. Select **Scripts & Plugins**. 4. Make sure the **Navigator** box is checked to **Enable JavaScript**. 5. Click **OK**.
Mozilla Firefox 1.4 or higher	1. Select **Tools → Options**. 2. Select the **Content** icon. 3. Select **Enable JavaScript**. 4. Click **OK**.

Set Cache to Always Reload a Page

Browser	Steps
Internet Explorer (IE) 6.0 or higher	1. Select **Tools → Internet Options**. 2. Select **General** tab. 3. Go to the **Temporary Internet Files** and click the **Settings** button. 4. Select the radio button for **Every visit to the page** and click **OK** when complete.
Netscape 7.1 or higher	1. Select **Edit → Preferences**. 2. Select **Advanced**. 3. Select **Cache**. 4. Select the **Every time I view the page** radio button. 5. Click **OK**.
Mozilla Firefox 1.4 or higher	1. Select **Tools → Options**. 2. Select the **Privacy** icon. 3. Click to expand Cache. 4. Set the value to "**0**" in the **Use up to: __ MB of disk space for the cache** field. 5. Click **OK**.

Plug-Ins

Adobe Acrobat Reader—With the free Acrobat Reader software, you can view and print Adobe PDF files. Many Evolve products offer student and instructor manuals, checklists, and more in this format!

Download at: http://www.adobe.com

Apple QuickTime—Install this to hear word pronunciations, heart and lung sounds, and many other helpful audio clips within Evolve Online Courses!

Download at: http://www.apple.com

Adobe Flash Player—This player will enhance your viewing of many Evolve web pages, as well as educational short-form to long-form animation within the Evolve Learning System!

Download at: http://www.adobe.com

Adobe Shockwave Player—Shockwave is best for viewing the many interactive learning activities within Evolve Online Courses!

Download at: http://www.adobe.com

Microsoft Word Viewer—With this viewer Microsoft Word users can share documents with those who don't have Word, and users without Word can open and view Word documents. Many Evolve products have testbank, student and instructor manuals, and other documents available for downloading and viewing on your own computer!

Download at: http://www.microsoft.com

Microsoft PowerPoint Viewer—View PowerPoint 97, 2000, and 2002 presentations even if you don't have PowerPoint with this viewer. Many Evolve products have slides available for downloading and viewing on your own computer!

Download at: http://www.microsoft.com

SUPPORT INFORMATION

Live support is available to customers in the United States and Canada from 7:30 a.m. to 7 p.m. (CST), Monday through Friday by calling **1-800-401-9962**. You can also send an email to evolve-support@elsevier.com.

There is also **24/7 support information** available on the Evolve website (http://evolve.elsevier.com), including:

- Guided Tours
- Tutorials
- Frequently Asked Questions (FAQs)
- Online Copies of Course User Guides
- And much more!

A QUICK TOUR

Welcome to *Virtual Clinical Excursions—Medical-Surgical*, a virtual hospital setting in which you can work with multiple complex patient simulations and also learn to access and evaluate the information resources that are essential for high-quality patient care.

The virtual hospital, Pacific View Regional Hospital, has realistic architecture and access to patient rooms, a Nurses' Station, and a Medication Room.

■ BEFORE YOU START

Make sure you have your textbook nearby when you use the *Virtual Clinical Excursions—Medical-Surgical* CD. You will want to consult topic areas in your textbook frequently while working with the CD and using this workbook.

■ HOW TO SIGN IN

- Enter your name on the Student Nurse identification badge.
- Now choose one of the four periods of care in which to work. In Periods of Care 1 through 3, you can actively engage in patient assessment, entry of data in the electronic patient record (EPR), and medication administration. Period of Care 4 presents the day in review. Highlight and click the appropriate period of care. (For this quick tour, choose **Period of Care 1: 0730-0815**.)
- This takes you to the Patient List screen (see example on page 11). Only the patients on the Medical-Surgical Floor are available. Note that the virtual time is provided in the box at the lower left corner of the screen (0730, since we chose Period of Care 1).

Note: If you choose to work during Period of Care 4: 1900-2000, the Patient List screen is skipped since you are not able to visit patients or administer medications during the shift. Instead, you are taken directly to the Nurses' Station, where the records of all the patients on the floor are available for your review.

■ **PATIENT LIST**

MEDICAL-SURGICAL UNIT

Harry George (Room 401)
Osteomyelitis—A 54-year-old Caucasian male admitted from a homeless shelter with an infected leg. He has complications of type 2 diabetes mellitus, alcohol abuse, nicotine addiction, poor pain control, and complex psychosocial issues.

Jacquline Catanazaro (Room 402)
Asthma—A 45-year-old Caucasian female admitted with an acute asthma exacerbation and suspected pneumonia. She has complications of chronic schizophrenia, noncompliance with medication therapy, obesity, and herniated disc.

Piya Jordan (Room 403)
Bowel obstruction—A 68-year-old Asian female admitted with a colon mass and suspected adenocarcinoma. She undergoes a right hemicolectomy. This patient's complications include atrial fibrillation, hypokalemia, and symptoms of meperidine toxicity.

Clarence Hughes (Room 404)
Degenerative joint disease—A 73-year-old African-American male admitted for a left total knee replacement. His preparations for discharge are complicated by the development of a pulmonary embolus and the need for ongoing intravenous therapy.

Pablo Rodriguez (Room 405)
Metastatic lung carcinoma—A 71-year-old Hispanic male admitted with symptoms of dehydration and malnutrition. He has chronic pain secondary to multiple subcutaneous skin nodules and psychosocial concerns related to family issues with his approaching death.

Patricia Newman (Room 406)
Pneumonia—A 61-year-old Caucasian female admitted with worsening pulmonary function and an acute respiratory infection. Her chronic emphysema is complicated by heavy smoking, hypertension, and malnutrition. She needs access to community resources such as a smoking cessation program and meal assistance.

■ HOW TO SELECT A PATIENT

- You can choose one or more patients to work with from the Patient List by checking the box to the left of the patient name(s). For this quick tour, select Piya Jordan and Pablo Rodriguez. (In order to receive a scorecard for a patient, the patient must be selected before proceeding to the Nurses' Station.)
- Click on **Get Report** to the right of the medical records number (MRN) to view a summary of the patient's care during the 12-hour period before your arrival on the unit.
- After reviewing the report, click on **Return to Patient List** and repeat the previous step to review the report of your second patient.
- When you are ready to begin your care, click on **Go to Nurses' Station** in the right lower corner.

Note: Even though the Patient List is initially skipped when you sign in to work for Period of Care 4, you can still access this screen if you wish to review the shift-change report for any of the patients. To do so, simply click on **Patient List** near the top left corner of the Nurses' Station (or click on the clipboard to the left of the Kardex). Then click on **Get Report** for the patient(s) whose care you are reviewing. This may be done during any period of care.

Virtual Clinical Excursions 3.0 : Medical Surgical Patient Set

Patient List

	Patient Name	Room	MRN	Clinical Report
☐	Harry George	401	1868054	Get Report
☐	Jacquline Catanazaro	402	1868048	Get Report
☑	Piya Jordan	403	1868092	Get Report
☐	Clarence Hughes	404	1868011	Get Report
☑	Pablo Rodriguez	405	1868088	Get Report
☐	Patricia Newman	406	1868097	Get Report

Please select all the patients you will be caring for this period of care. Once you have exited the patient list, you will not be able to change your current selections or select new patients to care for.

0730   Go to Nurses' Station

■ HOW TO FIND A PATIENT'S RECORDS

NURSES' STATION

Within the Nurses' Station, you will see:

1. A clipboard that contains the patient list for that floor.
2. A chart rack with patient charts labeled by room number, a notebook labeled Kardex, and a notebook labeled MAR (Medication Administration Record).
3. A desktop computer with access to the Electronic Patient Record (EPR).
4. A tool bar across the top of the screen that can also be used to access the Patient List, EPR, Chart, MAR, and Kardex. This tool bar is also accessible from each patient's room.
5. A Drug Guide containing information about the medications you are able to administer to your patients.
6. A tool bar across the bottom of the screen that you can use to access patient rooms, the Medication Room, the Floor Map, or the Drug Guide.

As you run your cursor over an item, it will be highlighted. To select, simply double-click on the item. As you use these resources, you will always be able to return to the Nurses' Station by clicking on the **Return to Nurses' Station** bar located in the right lower corner of your screen.

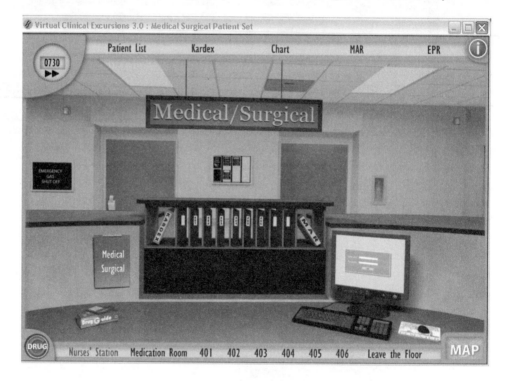

MEDICATION ADMINISTRATION RECORD (MAR)

The MAR icon located in the tool bar at the top of your screen accesses current 24-hour medications for each patient. Click on the icon and the MAR will open. (*Note:* You can also access the MAR by clicking on the MAR notebook on the far right side of the book rack in the center of the screen.) Within the MAR, tabs on the right side of the screen allow you to select patients by room number. Be careful to make sure you select the correct tab number for *your* patient rather than simply reading the first record that appears after the MAR opens. Each MAR sheet lists the following:

- Medications
- Route and dosage of each medication
- Times of administration of each medication

Note: The MAR changes each day. Expired MARs are stored in the patients' charts.

CHARTS

To access patient charts, either click on the **Chart** icon at the top of your screen or anywhere within the chart rack in the center of the Nurses' Station screen. When the close-up view appears, the individual charts are labeled by room number. To open a chart, click on the room number of the patient whose chart you wish to review. The patient's name and allergies will appear on the left side of the screen, along with a list of tabs on the right side of the screen, allowing you to view the following data:

- Allergies
- Physician's Orders
- Physician's Notes
- Nurse's Notes
- Laboratory Reports
- Diagnostic Reports
- Surgical Reports
- Consultations

- Patient Education
- History and Physical
- Nursing Admission
- Expired MARs
- Consents
- Mental Health
- Admissions
- Emergency Department

Information appears in real time. The entries are in reverse chronologic order, so use the down arrow at the right side of each chart page to scroll down to view previous entries. Flip from tab to tab to view multiple data fields or click on the **Return to Nurses' Station** bar in the lower right corner of the screen to exit the chart.

ELECTRONIC PATIENT RECORD (EPR)

The EPR can be accessed from the computer in the Nurses' Station or from the EPR icon located in the tool bar at the top of your screen. To access a patient's EPR:
- Click on either the computer screen or the **EPR** icon.
- Your username and password are automatically filled in.
- Click on **Login** to enter the EPR.
- *Note:* Like the MAR, the EPR is arranged numerically. Thus when you enter, you are initially shown the records of the patient in the lowest room number on the floor. To view the correct data for *your* patient, remember to select the correct room number, using the drop-down menu for the Patient field at the top left corner of the screen.

The EPR used in Pacific View Regional Hospital represents a composite of commercial versions being used in hospitals. You can access the EPR:
- to review existing data for a patient (by room number).
- to enter data you collect while working with a patient.

The EPR is updated daily, so no matter what day or part of a shift you are working, there will be a current EPR with the patient's data from the past days of the current hospital stay. This type of simulated EPR allows you to examine how data for different attributes have changed over time, as well as to examine data for all of a patient's attributes at a particular time. The EPR is fully functional (as it is in a real-life hospital). You can enter such data as blood pressure, breath sounds, and certain treatments. The EPR will not, however, allow you to enter data for a previous time period. Use the arrows at the bottom of the screen to move forward and backward in time.

Virtual Clinical Excursions 3.0 : Medical Surgical Patient Set				
Patient: 403 **Category:** Vital Signs				**0732**
Name: Piya Jordan	Wed 0630	Wed 0700	Wed 0715	Code Meanings
PAIN: LOCATION		OS		A Abdomen
PAIN: RATING		5		Ar Arm
PAIN: CHARACTERISTICS		C		B Back
PAIN: VOCAL CUES		VC3		C Chest
PAIN: FACIAL CUES		FC1		Ft Foot
PAIN: BODILY CUES				H Head
PAIN: SYSTEM CUES				Hd Hand
PAIN: FUNCTIONAL EFFECTS				L Left
PAIN: PREDISPOSING FACTORS				Lg Leg
PAIN: RELIEVING FACTORS				Lw Lower
PCA		P		N Neck
TEMPERATURE (F)		99.6		NN See Nurses notes
TEMPERATURE (C)				OS Operative site
MODE OF MEASUREMENT		Ty		Or See Physicians orders
SYSTOLIC PRESSURE		110		PN See Progress notes
DIASTOLIC PRESSURE		70		R Right
BP MODE OF MEASUREMENT		NIBP		Up Upper
HEART RATE		104		
RESPIRATORY RATE		18		
SpO2 (%)		95		
BLOOD GLUCOSE				
WEIGHT				
HEIGHT				
	◄		►	Exit EPR

At the top of the EPR screen, you can choose patients by their room numbers. In addition, you have access to 17 different categories of patient data. To change patients or data categories, click the down arrow to the right of the room number or category.

The categories of patient data in the EPR as as follows:

- Vital Signs
- Respiratory
- Cardiovascular
- Neurologic
- Gastrointestinal
- Excretory
- Musculoskeletal
- Integumentary
- Reproductive
- Psychosocial
- Wounds and Drains
- Activity
- Hygiene and Comfort
- Safety
- Nutrition
- IV
- Intake and Output

Remember, each hospital selects its own codes. The codes used in the EPR at Pacific View Regional Hospital may be different from ones you have seen in your clinical rotations. Take some time to acquaint yourself with the codes. Within the Vital Signs category, click on any item in the left column (e.g., Pain: Characteristics). In the far-right column, you will see a list of code meanings for the possible findings and/or descriptors for that assessment area.

You will use the codes to record the data you collect as you work with patients. Click on the box in the last time column to the right of any item and wait for the code meanings applicable to that entry to appear. Select the appropriate code to describe your assessment findings and type it in the box. (*Note:* If no cursor appears within the box, click on the box again until the blue shading disappears and the blinking cursor appears.) Once the data are typed in this box, they are entered into the patient's record for this period of care only.

To leave the EPR, click on **Exit EPR** in the bottom right corner of the screen.

■ **VISITING A PATIENT**

From the Nurses' Station, click on the room number of the patient you wish to visit in the tool bar at the bottom of your screen. Once you are inside the room, you will see a still photo of your patient in the top left corner. To verify that this is the patient you have chosen, click on the **Check Armband** icon to the right of the photo. The patient's identification data will appear. If you click on **Check Allergies** (the next icon to the right), a list of the patient's allergies (if any) will replace the photo.

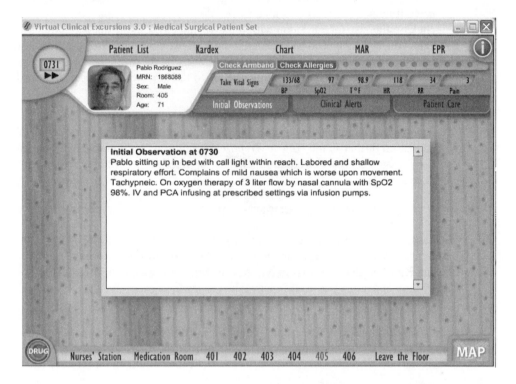

Also located in the patient's room are multiple icons you can use to assess the patient or the patient's medications. A virtual clock is provided in the upper left corner of the room to monitor your progress in real time. (*Note:* The fast-forward icon within the virtual clock will advance the time by 2-minute intervals when clicked.)

- The tool bar across the top of the screen allows you to check the **Patient List**, access the **EPR** to check or enter data, and view the patient's **Chart**, **MAR**, or **Kardex**.

- The **Take Vital Signs** icon allows you to measure the patient's up-to-the-minute blood pressure, oxygen saturation, temperature, heart rate, respiratory rate, and pain level.

- Each time you enter a patient's room, you are given an Initial Observation report to review (in the text box under the patient's photo). These notes are provided to give you a "look" at the patient as if you had just stepped into the room. You can also click on the **Initial Observations** icon to return to this box from other views within the patient's room. To the right of this icon is **Clinical Alerts**, a resource that allows you to make decisions about priority medication interventions based on emerging data collected in real time. Check this screen throughout your period of care to avoid missing critical information related to recently ordered or STAT medications.

- Clicking on the **Patient Care** icon opens up three specific learning environments within the patient room: **Physical Assessment**, **Nurse-Client Interactions**, and **Medication Administration**.

- To perform a **Physical Assessment**, choose a body area (such as **Head & Neck**) by clicking on the appropriate icon in the column of yellow buttons. This activates a list of system subcategories for that body area (e.g., see **Sensory**, **Neurologic**, etc. in the green boxes). After you click on the system that you wish to evaluate, a still photo and text box appear, describing the assessment findings. The still photo is a "snapshot" of how an assessment of this area might be done or what the finding might look like. For every body area, there is also an **Equipment** button located on the far right of the screen.

- To the right of the Physical Assessment icon is **Nurse-Client Interactions**. Clicking on this icon will reveal the times and titles of any videos available for viewing. (*Note:* If the video you wish to see is not listed, this means you have not yet reached the correct virtual time to view that video. Check the virtual clock; you may return to access the video once its designated time has occurred—as long as you do so within the same period of care. Or you can click on the fast-forward icon within the virtual clock to advance the time by 2-minute intervals. You will then need to click again on **Patient Care** and **Nurse-Client Interactions** to refresh the screen.) To view a listed video, click on the white arrow to the right of the video title. Use the control buttons below the video to start, stop, pause, rewind, or fast-forward the action or to mute the sound.

- **Medication Administration** is the pathway that allows you to review and administer medications to a patient after you have prepared them in the Medication Room. This process is addressed further in the *How to Prepare Medications* section (pages 19-20) and in *Medications* (pages 26-30). For additional hands-on practice, see *Reducing Medication Errors* (pages 37-41).

■ HOW TO QUIT, CHANGE PATIENTS, OR CHANGE PERIOD OF CARE

How to Quit: From most screens, you may click the **Leave the Floor** icon on the bottom tool bar to the right of the patient room numbers. (*Note:* From some screens, you will first need to click an **Exit** button or **Return to Nurses' Station** before clicking **Leave the Floor**.) When the Floor Menu appears, click **Exit** to leave the program.

How to Change Patients or Period of Care: To change patients, simply click on the new patient's room number. (You cannot receive a scorecard for a new patient, however, unless you have already selected that patient on the Patient List screen.) To change to a new period of care or to restart the virtual clock, click on **Leave the Floor** and then on **Restart the Program**.

Virtual Clinical Excursions 3.0 : Medical Surgical Patient Set

Floor Menu

Look at your Preceptor's Evaluation.
Evaluations provide feedback on the work you completed during patient care. If you choose the Preceptor's Evaluation you will no longer be able to return to the floor.

Take a break.
Time will be stopped until you wish to return to the simulation.

Restart the program.
If you restart, all data from your work in the current Period of Care will be erased.

CREDITS View Credits
Take a look at the list of professionals who took part in the creation of this software suite.

EXIT Exit the program.
If you choose to exit, all data from your work within the current Period of Care will be erased.

0732   Return to Room 405

■ HOW TO PREPARE MEDICATIONS

From the Nurses' Station or the patient's room, you can access the Medication Room by clicking on the icon in the tool bar at the bottom of your screen to the left of the patient room numbers.

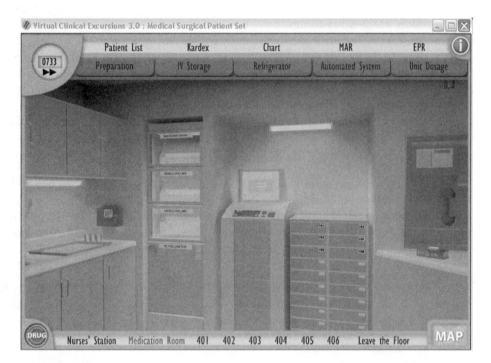

In the Medication Room you have access to the following (from left to right):

- A preparation area is located on the counter under the cabinets. To begin the medication preparation process, click on the tray on the counter or click on the **Preparation** icon at the top of the screen. The next screen leads you through a specific sequence (called the Preparation Wizard) to prepare medications one at a time for administration to a patient. However, no medication has been selected at this time. We will do this while working with a patient in *A Detailed Tour*. To exit this screen, click on **View Medication Room**.

- To the right of the cabinets (and above the refrigerator), IV storage bins are provided. Click on the bins themselves or on the **IV Storage** icon at the top of the screen. The bins are labeled **Microinfusion**, **Small Volume**, and **Large Volume**. Click on an individual bin to see a list of its contents. If you needed to prepare an IV medication at this time, you could click on the medication and its label would appear to the right under the patient's name. Next, you would click **Put Medication on Tray**. If you ever change your mind or choose the incorrect medication, you can reverse your actions by clicking on **Put Medication in Bin**. Click **Close Bin** in the right bottom corner to exit. **View Medication Room** brings you back to a full view of the entire room.

- A refrigerator is located under the IV storage bins to hold any medications that must be stored below room temperature. Click on the refrigerator door or on the **Refrigerator** icon at the top of the screen. Then click on the close-up view of the door to access the medications. When you are finished, click **Close Door** and then **View Medication Room**.

- To prepare controlled substances, click the **Automated System** icon at the top of the screen or click the computer monitor located to the right of the IV storage bins. A login screen will appear; your name and password are automatically filled in. Click **Login**. Select the patient for whom you wish to access medications; then select the correct medication drawer to open (they are stored alphabetically). Click **Open Drawer**, highlight the proper medication, and choose **Put Medication on Tray**. When you are finished, click **Close Drawer** and then **View Medication Room**.

- Next to the Automated System is a set of drawers identified by patient room number. To access these, click on the drawers themselves or on the **Unit Dosage** icon at the top of the screen. This provides a close-up view of the drawers. To open a drawer, click on the room number of the patient you are working with. Next, click on the medication you would like to prepare for the patient, and a label will appear to the right, listing the medication strength, units, and dosage per unit. You can **Open** and **Close** this medication label by clicking the appropriate icon. To exit, click **Close Drawer**; then click **View Medication Room**.

At any time, you can learn about a medication you wish to prepare for a patient by clicking on the **Drug** icon in the bottom left corner of the medication room screen or by clicking the **Drug Guide** book on the counter to the right of the unit dosage drawers. The **Drug Guide** provides information about the medications commonly included in nursing drug handbooks. Nutritional supplements and maintenance intravenous fluid preparations are not included.

To access the MAR to review the medications ordered for a patient, click on the **MAR** icon located in the tool bar at the top of your screen and then click on the correct tab for your patient's room number. You may also click the **Review MAR** icon in the tool bar at the bottom of your screen from inside each medication storage area.

After you have chosen and prepared your medications, return to the patient's room to administer them by clicking on the room number in the bottom tool bar. Once inside the patient's room, click on **Patient Care** and then on **Medication Administration** and follow the proper administration sequence.

■ PRECEPTOR'S EVALUATIONS

When you have finished a session, click on **Leave the Floor** to go to the Floor Menu. At this point, you can click on the top icon (**Look at Your Preceptor's Evaluation**) to receive a score-card that provides feedback on the work you completed during patient care.

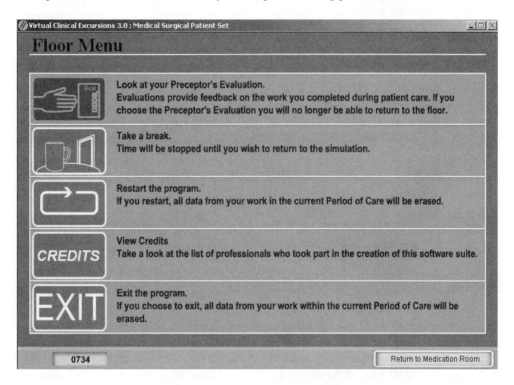

Evaluations are available for each patient you selected when you signed in for the current period of care. Click on the **Medication Scorecard** icon to see an example.

The scorecard compares the medications you administered to a patient during a period of care with what should have been administered. Table A lists the correct medications. Table B lists any medications that were administered incorrectly.

Remember, not every medication listed on the MAR should necessarily be given. For example, a patient might have an allergy to a drug that was ordered, or a medication might have been improperly transcribed to the MAR. Predetermined medication "errors" embedded within the program challenge you to exercise critical thinking skills and professional judgment when deciding to administer a medication, just as you would in a real hospital. Use all your available resources, such as the patient's chart and the MAR, to make your decision.

Table C lists the resources that were available to assist you in medication administration. It also documents whether and when you accessed these resources. For example, did you check the patient armband or perform a check of vital signs? If so, when?

You can click **Print** to get a copy of this report if needed. When you have finished reviewing the scorecard, click **Return to Evaluations** and then **Return to Menu**.

■ FLOOR MAP

To get a general sense of your location within the hospital, you can click on the **Map** icon found in the lower right corner of most of the screens in the *Virtual Clinical Excursions—Medical-Surgical* program. (*Note:* If you are following this quick tour step by step, you will need to **Restart the Program** from the Floor Menu, sign in again, and go to the Nurses' Station to access the map.) When you click the **Map** icon, a floor map appears, showing the layout of the floor you are currently on, as well as a directory of the patients and services on that floor. As you move your cursor over the directory list, the location of each room is highlighted on the map (and vice versa). The floor map can be accessed from the Nurses' Station, Medication Room, and each patient's room.

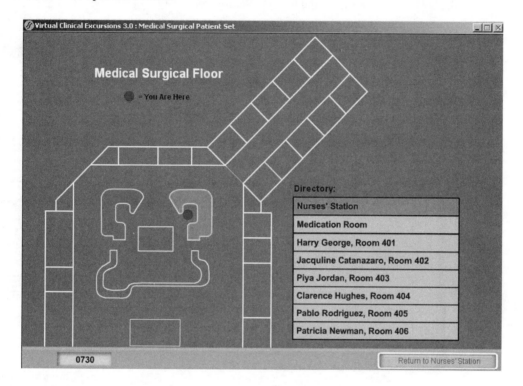

A DETAILED TOUR

If you wish to more thoroughly understand the capabilities of *Virtual Clinical Excursions—Medical-Surgical*, take a detailed tour by completing the following section. During this tour, we will work with a specific patient to introduce you to all the different components and learning opportunities available within the software.

■ WORKING WITH A PATIENT

Sign in for Period of Care 1 (0730-0815). From the Patient List, select Piya Jordan in Room 403; however, do not go to the Nurses' Station yet.

■ REPORT

In hospitals, when one shift ends and another begins, the outgoing nurse who attended a patient will give a verbal and sometimes a written summary of that patient's condition to the incoming nurse who will assume care for the patient. This summary is called a report and is an important source of data to provide an overview of a patient. Your first task is to get the clinical report on Piya Jordan. To do this, click **Get Report** in the far right column in this patient's row. From a brief review of this summary, identify the problems and areas of concern that you will need to address for this patient.

When you have finished noting any areas of concern, click **Go to Nurses' Station**.

■ CHARTS

You can access Piya Jordan's chart from the Nurses' Station or from the patient's room (403). We will access it from the Nurses' Station: Click on the chart rack or on the **Chart** icon in the tool bar at the top of your screen. Next, click on the chart labeled **403** to open the medical record for Piya Jordan. Click on the **Emergency Department** tab to view a record of why this patient was admitted.

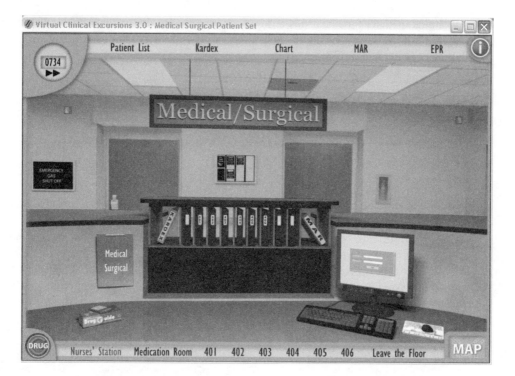

How many days has Piya Jordan been in the hospital?

What tests were done upon her arrival in the Emergency Department and why?

What was her reason for admission?

You should also click on **Surgical Reports** to learn what procedures were performed and when. Finally, review the **Nursing Admission** and **History and Physical** to learn about the health history of this patient. When you are done reviewing the chart, click **Return to Nurses' Station**.

■ MEDICATIONS

Open the Medication Administration Record (MAR) by clicking on the **MAR** icon in the tool bar at the top of your screen. *Remember:* The MAR automatically opens to the first occupied room number on the floor—which is not necessarily your patient's room number! Since you need to access Piya Jordan's MAR, click on tab **403** (her room number). Always make sure you are giving the *Right Drug to the Right Patient!*

Examine the list of medications ordered for Piya Jordan. In the table below, list the medications that need to be given during this period of care (0730-0815). For each medication, note the dosage, route, and time to be given.

Time	Medication	Dosage	Route

Click on **Return to Nurses' Station**. Next, click on **403** on the bottom tool bar and then verify that you are indeed in Piya Jordan's room. Select **Clinical Alerts** (the icon to the right of Initial Observations) to check for any emerging data that might affect your medication administration priorities. Next, go to the patient's chart (click on the **Chart** icon; then click on **403**). When the chart opens, select the **Physician's Orders** tab.

Review the orders. Have any new medications been ordered? Return to the MAR (click **Return to Room 403**; then click **MAR**). Verify that the new medications have been correctly transcribed to the MAR. Mistakes are sometimes made in the transcription process in the hospital setting, and it is sound practice to double-check any new order.

Are there any patient assessments you will need to perform before administering these medications? If so, return to Room 403 and click on **Patient Care** and then **Physical Assessment** to complete those assessments before proceeding.

Now click on the **Medication Room** icon in the tool bar at the bottom of your screen to locate and prepare the medications for Piya Jordan.

In the Medication Room, you must access the medications for Piya Jordan from the specific dispensing system in which each medication is stored. Locate each medication that needs to be given in this time period and click on **Put Medication on Tray** as appropriate. (*Hint:* Look in Unit Dosage drawer first.) When you are finished, click on **Close Drawer** and then on **View Medication Room**. Now click on the medication tray on the counter on the left side of the medication room screen to begin preparing the medications you have selected. (*Remember:* You can also click **Preparation** in the tool bar at the top of the screen.)

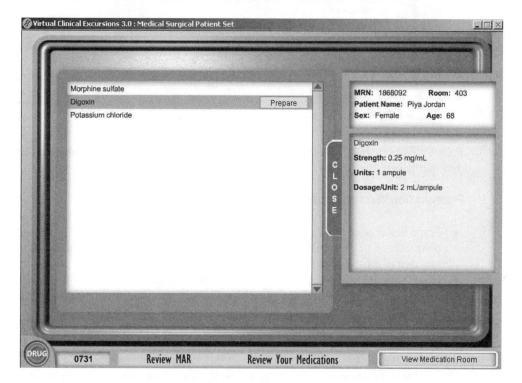

In the preparation area, you should see a list of the medications you put on the tray in the previous steps. Click on the first medication and then click **Prepare**. Follow the onscreen instructions of the Preparation Wizard, providing any data requested. As an example, let's follow the preparation process for digoxin, one of the medications due to be administered to Piya Jordan during this period of care. To begin, click to select **Digoxin**; then click **Prepare**. Now work through the Preparation Wizard sequence as detailed below:

> Amount of medication in the ampule: 2 mL.
> Enter the amount of medication you will draw up into a syringe: **0.5** mL.
> Click **Next**.
> Select the patient you wish to set aside the medication for: **Room 403, Piya Jordan**.
> Click **Finish**.
> Click **Return to Medication Room**.

Follow this same basic process for the other medications due to be administered to Piya Jordan during this period of care. (*Hint:* Look in **IV Storage** and **Automated System**.)

PREPARATION WIZARD EXCEPTIONS

- Some medications in *Virtual Clinical Excursions—Medical-Surgical* are preprepared by the pharmacy (e.g., IV antibiotics) and taken to the patient room as a whole. This is common practice in most hospitals.
- Blood products are not administered by students through the *Virtual Clinical Excursions—Medical-Surgical* simulations since blood administration follows specific protocols not covered in this program.
- The *Virtual Clinical Excursions—Medical-Surgical* simulations do not allow for mixing more than one type of medication, such as regular and Lente insulins, in the same syringe. In the clinical setting, when multiple types of insulin are ordered for a patient, the regular insulin is drawn up first, followed by the longer-acting insulin. Insulin is always administered in a special unit-marked syringe.

Now return to Room 403 (click on **403** on the bottom tool bar) to administer Piya Jordan's medications.

At any time during the medication administration process, you can perform a further review of systems, take vital signs, check information contained within the chart, or verify patient identity and allergies. Inside Piya Jordan's room, click **Take Vital Signs**. (*Note:* These findings change over time to reflect the temporal changes you would find in a patient similar to Piya Jordan.)

When you have gathered all the data you need, click on **Patient Care** and then select **Medication Administration**. Any medications you prepared in the previous steps should be listed on the left side of your screen. Let's continue the administration process with the digoxin ordered for Piya Jordan. Click to highlight **Digoxin** in the list of medications. Next, click on the down arrow to the right of **Select** and choose **Administer** from the drop-down menu. This will activate the Administration Wizard. Complete the Wizard sequence as follows:

- Route: **IV**
- Method: **Direct Injection**
- Site: **Peripheral IV**
- Click **Administer to Patient** arrow.
- Would you like to document this administration in the MAR? **Yes**
- Click **Finish** arrow.

Your selections are recorded by a tracking system and evaluated on a Medication Scorecard stored under Preceptor's Evaluations. This scorecard can be viewed, printed, and given to your instructor. To access the Preceptor's Evaluations, click on **Leave the Floor**. When the Floor Menu appears, click on the icon next to **Look at Your Preceptor's Evaluation**. Then click on **Medication Scorecard** inside the box with Piya Jordan's name (see example on the following page).

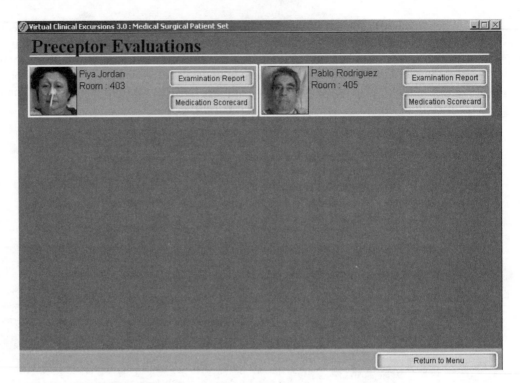

■ MEDICATION SCORECARD

- First, review Table A. Was digoxin given correctly? Did you give the other medications as ordered?
- Table B shows you which (if any) medications you gave incorrectly.
- Table C addresses the resources used for Piya Jordan. Did you access the patient's chart, MAR, EPR, or Kardex as needed to make safe medication administration decisions?
- Did you check the patient's armband to verify her identity? Did you check whether your patient had any known allergies to medications? Were vital signs taken?

When you have finished reviewing the scorecard, click **Return to Evaluations** and then **Return to Menu**.

■ **VITAL SIGNS**

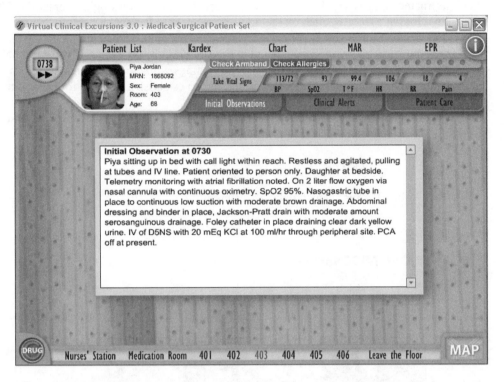

Vital signs, often considered the traditional "signs of life," include body temperature, heart rate, respiratory rate, blood pressure, oxygen saturation of the blood, and pain level.

Inside Piya Jordan's room, click **Take Vital Signs**. (*Note:* If you are following this detailed tour step by step, you will need to **Restart the Program** from the Floor Menu, sign in again, and navigate to Room 403.) Collect vital signs for this patient and record them in the following table. Note the time at which you collected each of these data. (*Remember:* You can take vital signs at any time. The data change over time to reflect the temporal changes you would find in a patient similar to Piya Jordan.)

Vital Signs	Findings/Time
Blood pressure	
O$_2$ saturation	
Heart rate	
Respiratory rate	
Temperature	
Pain rating	

After you are done, click on the **EPR** icon located in the tool bar at the top of the screen. Your username and password are automatically provided. Click on **Login** to enter the EPR. To access Piya Jordan's records, click on the down arrow next to Patient and choose her room number, **403**. Select **Vital Signs** as the category. Next, in the empty time column on the far right, record the vital signs data you just collected in Piya Jordan's room. (*Note:* If you need help with this process, see page 16.) Now compare these findings with the data you collected earlier for this patient's vital signs. Use these earlier findings to establish a baseline for each of the vital signs.

    a.   Are any of the data you collected significantly different from the baseline for a particular vital sign?

         Circle One: Yes   No

    b.   If "Yes," which data are different?

■ PHYSICAL ASSESSMENT

After you have finished examining the EPR for vital signs, click **Exit EPR** to return to Room 403. Click **Patient Care** and then **Physical Assessment**. Think about what information you received in the report at the beginning of this shift, as well as what you may have learned about this patient from the chart. Based on this, what area(s) of examination should you pay most attention to at this time? Is there any equipment you should be monitoring? Conduct a physical assessment of the body areas and systems that you consider priorities for Piya Jordan. For example, select **Head & Neck**; then click on and assess **Sensory** and **Lymphatic**. Complete any other assessment(s) you think are necessary at this time. In the following table, record the data you collected during this examination.

Area of Examination	Findings
Head & Neck Sensory	
Head & Neck Lymphatic	

After you have finished collecting these data, return to the EPR. Compare the data that were already in the record with those you just collected.

    a.   Are any of the data you collected significantly different from the baselines for this patient?

        Circle One: Yes   No

    b.   If "Yes," which data are different?

■ NURSE-CLIENT INTERACTIONS

Click on **Patient Care** from inside Piya Jordan's room (403). Now click on **Nurse-Client Interactions** to access a short video titled **Pain—Adverse Drug Event**, which is available for viewing at or after 0735 (based on the virtual clock in the upper left corner of your screen; see *Note* below). To begin the video, click on the arrow next to its title. You will observe a nurse communicating with Piya Jordan and her daughter. There are many variations of nursing practice, some exemplifying "best" practice and some not. Note whether the nurse in this interaction displays professional behavior and compassionate care. Are her words congruent with what is going on with the patient? Does this interaction "feel right" to you? If not, how would you handle this situation differently? Explain.

Note: If the video you wish to view is not listed, this means you have not yet reached the correct virtual time to view that video. Check the virtual clock; you may return to access the video once its designated time has occurred—as long as you do so within the same period of care. Or you can click on the fast-forward icon within the virtual clock to advance the time by 2-minute intervals. You will then need to click again on **Patient Care** and **Nurse-Client Interactions** to refresh the screen.

At least one Nurse-Client Interactions video is available during each period of care. Viewing these videos can help you learn more about what is occurring with a patient at a certain time and also prompt you to discern between nurse communications that are ideal and those that need improvement. Compassionate care and the ability to communicate clearly are essential components of delivering quality nursing care, and it is during your clinical time that you will begin to refine these skills.

■ COLLECTING AND EVALUATING DATA

Each of the activities you perform in the Patient Care environment generates a significant amount of assessment data. Remember that after you collect data, you can record your findings in the EPR. You can also review the EPR, patient's chart, videos, and MAR at any time. You will get plenty of practice collecting and then evaluating data in context of the patient's course.

Now, here's an important question for you:

> Did the previous sequence of exercises provide the most efficient way to assess Piya Jordan?

For example, you went to the patient's room to get vital signs, then back to the EPR to enter data and compare your findings with extant data. Next, you went back to the patient's room to do a physical examination, then again back to the EPR to enter and review data. If this back-and-forth process of data collection and recording seemed inefficient, remember the following:

- Plan all of your nursing activities to maximize efficiency, while at the same time optimizing the quality of patient care. (Think about what data you might need before performing certain tasks. For example, do you need to check a heart rate before administering a cardiac medication or check an IV site before starting an infusion?)

- You collect a tremendous amount of data when you work with a patient. Very few people can accurately remember all these data for more than a few minutes. Develop efficient assessment skills, and record data as soon as possible after collecting them.

- Assessment data are only the starting point for the nursing process.

Make a clear distinction between these first exercises and how you actually provide nursing care. These initial exercises were designed to involve you actively in the use of different software components. This workbook focuses on sensible practices for implementing the nursing process in ways that ensure the highest-quality care of patients.

Most important, remember that a human being changes through time, and that these changes include both the physical and psychosocial facets of a person as a living organism. Think about this for a moment. Some patients may change physically in a very short time (a patient with emerging myocardial infarction) or more slowly (a patient with a chronic illness). Patients' overall physical and psychosocial conditions may improve or deteriorate. They may have effective coping skills and familial support, or they may feel alone and full of despair. In fact, each individual is a complex mix of physical and psychosocial elements, and at least some of these elements usually change through time.

Thus it is crucial that you *DO NOT* think of the nursing process as a simple one-time, five-step procedure consisting of assessment, nursing diagnosis, planning, implementation, and evaluation. Rather, the nursing process should be utilized as a creative and systematic approach to delivering nursing care. Furthermore, because all living organisms are constantly changing, we must apply the nursing process over and over. Each time we follow the nursing process for an individual patient, we refine our understanding of that patient's physical and psychosocial conditions based on collection and analysis of many different types of data. *Virtual Clinical Excursions—Medical-Surgical* will help you develop both the creativity and the systematic approach needed to become a nurse who is equipped to deliver the highest-quality care to all patients.

REDUCING MEDICATION ERRORS

Earlier in this detailed tour, you learned the basic steps of medication preparation and administration. The following simulations will allow you to practice those skills further—with an increased emphasis on reducing medication errors by using the Medication Scorecard to evaluate your work.

Sign in to work at Pacific View Regional Hospital for Period of Care 1. (*Note:* If you are already working with another patient or during another period of care, click on **Leave the Floor** and then **Restart the Program**; then sign in.)

From the Patient List, select Clarence Hughes. Then click on **Go to Nurses' Station**. Complete the following steps to prepare and administer medications to Clarence Hughes.

- Click on **Medication Room**.
- Click on **MAR** and then on tab **404** to determine prn medications that have been ordered for Clarence Hughes to address his constipation and pain. (*Note:* You may click on **Review MAR** at any time to verify the correct medication order. Always remember to check the patient name on the MAR to make sure you have the correct patient's record—you must click on the correct room number tab within the MAR.) Click on **Return to Medication Room** after reviewing the correct MAR.
- Click on **Unit Dosage** (or on the Unit Dosage cabinet); from the close-up view, click on drawer **404**.
- Select the medications you would like to administer. After each selection, click **Put Medication on Tray**. When you are finished selecting medications, click **Close Drawer** and then **View Medication Room**.
- Click on **Automated System** (or on the Automated System unit itself). Click **Login**.
- On the next screen, specify the correct patient and drawer location.
- Select the medication you would like to administer and click on **Put Medication on Tray**. Repeat this process if you wish to administer other medications from the Automated System.
- When you are finished, click **Close Drawer** and **View Medication Room**.
- From the Medication Room, click on **Preparation** (or on the preparation tray).
- From the list of medications on your tray, highlight the correct medication to administer and click **Prepare**.
- This activates the Preparation Wizard. Supply any requested information; then click **Next**.
- Now select the correct patient to receive this medication and click **Finish**.
- Repeat the previous three steps until all medications that you want to administer are prepared.
- You can click on **Review Your Medications** and then on **Return to Medication Room** when ready. Once you are back in the Medication Room, go directly to Clarence Hughes' room by clicking on **404** at bottom of screen.
- Inside the patient's room, administer the medication, utilizing the five rights of medication administration. After you have collected the appropriate assessment data and are ready for administration, click **Patient Care** and then **Medication Administration**. Verify that the correct patient and medication(s) appear in the left-hand window. Highlight the first medication you wish to administer; then click the down arrow next to Select. From the drop-down menu, select **Administer** and complete the Administration Wizard by providing any information requested. When the Wizard stops asking for information, click **Administer to Patient**. Specify **Yes** when asked whether this administration should be recorded in the MAR. Finally, click **Finish**.

■ **SELF-EVALUATION**

Now let's see how you did during your medication administration!

- Click on **Leave the Floor** at the bottom of your screen. From the Floor Menu, select **Look at Your Preceptor's Evaluation**. Then click on **Medication Scorecard** for Clarence Hughes. These resources will help you find out more about each patient's medications and possible sources of medication errors.

1. Start by examining Table A. These are the medications you should have given to Clarence Hughes during this period of care. If each of the medications in Table A has a √ by it, then you made no errors. Congratulations!

If any medication has an X by it, then you made one or more medication errors.

Compare Tables A and B to determine which of the following types of errors you made: Wrong Dose, Wrong Route/Method/Site, or Wrong Time. Follow these steps:
   a. Find medications in Table A that were given incorrectly.
   b. Now see if those same medications are in Table B, which shows what you actually administered to Clarence Hughes.
   c. Comparing Tables A and B, match the Strength, Dose, Route/Method/Site, and Time for each medication you administered incorrectly.
   d. Then, using the form below, list the medications given incorrectly and mark the errors you made for each medication.

Medication	Strength	Dosage	Route	Method	Site	Time
	❑	❑	❑	❑	❑	❑
	❑	❑	❑	❑	❑	❑
	❑	❑	❑	❑	❑	❑
	❑	❑	❑	❑	❑	❑

2. To help you reduce future medication errors, consider the following list of possible reasons for errors.

   - Did not check drug against MAR for correct patient, correct date, correct time, correct drug, and correct dose.
   - Did not check drug dose against MAR three times.
   - Did not open the unit dose package in the patient's room.
   - Did not correctly identify the patient using two identifiers.
   - Did not administer the drug on time.
   - Did not verify patient allergies.
   - Did not check the patient's current condition or vital sign parameters.
   - Did not consider why the patient would be receiving this drug.
   - Did not question why the drug was in the patient's drawer.
   - Did not check the physician's order and/or check with the pharmacist when there was a question about the drug or dose.
   - Did not verify that no adverse effects had occurred from a previous dose.

Based on these possibilities, determine how you made each error and record the reason into the form below:

Medication	Reason for Error

3. Look again at Table B. Are there medications listed that are not in Table A? If so, you gave a medication to Clarence Hughes that he should not have received. Complete the following exercises to help you understand how such an error might have been made.

   a. Perhaps you gave a medication that was on Clarence Hughes' MAR for this period of care, without recognizing that a change had occurred in the patient's condition, which should have caused you to reconsider. Review patient records as necessary and complete the following form:

Medication	Possible Reasons Not to Give This Medication

   b. Another possibility is that you gave Clarence Hughes a medication that should have been given at a different time. Check his MAR and complete the form below to determine whether you made a Wrong Time error:

Medication	Given to Clarence Hughes at What Time	Should Have Been Given at What Time

c. Maybe you gave another patient's medication to Clarence Hughes. In this case, you made a Wrong Patient error. Check the MARs of other patients and use the form below to determine whether you made this type of error:

Medication	Given to Clarence Hughes	Should Have Been Given to

4. The Medication Scorecard provides some other interesting sources of information. For example, if there is a medication selected for Clarence Hughes but it was not given to him, there will be an X by that medication in Table A, but it will not appear in Table B. In that case, you might have given this medication to some other patient, which is another type of Wrong Patient error. To investigate further, look at Table D, which lists the medications you gave to other patients. See whether you can find any medications for Clarence Hughes that were given to another patient by mistake. However, before you make any decisions, be sure to cross-check the MAR for other patients because the same medication may have been ordered for multiple patients. Use the following form to record your findings:

Medication	Should Have Been Given to Clarence Hughes	Given by Mistake to

5. Now take some time to review the medication exercises you just completed. Use the form below to create an overall analysis of what you have learned. Once again, record each of the medication errors you made, including the type of each error. Then, for each error you made, indicate specifically what you would do differently to prevent this type of error from occurring again.

Medication	Type of Error	Error Prevention Tactic

Submit this form to your instructor if required as a graded assignment, or simply use these exercises to improve your understanding of medication errors and how to reduce them.

Name: _____   Date: _____

The following icons are used throughout the workbook to help you quickly identify particular activities and assignments:

 Indicates a reading assignment—tells you which textbook chapter(s) you should read before starting each lesson

 Indicates a writing activity

 Marks the beginning of an interactive CD-ROM activity—signals you to open or return to your *Virtual Clinical Excursions—Medical-Surgical* CD-ROM

 Indicates additional CD-ROM instructions

 Indicates questions and activities that require you to consult your textbook

Indicates the approximate time required to complete an exercise

LESSON **1** _____

Cultural Aspects of Health

_____

/O̶R̶O̶ **Reading Assignment:** Cultural Aspects of Health (Chapter 6)

Patients: Piya Jordan, Room 403
Clarence Hughes, Room 404
Pablo Rodriguez, Room 405

Goal: Demonstrate understanding and appropriate application of cultural concepts related to health care.

Objectives:

1. Define *cultural competence* and *culture*.
2. Identify appropriate methods of assessing the culture of a patient.
3. Identify specific needs for patients of various cultural backgrounds.
4. Describe nursing interventions relevant for patients of various cultures.
5. Correctly utilize the nursing process in providing culturally competent nursing care.

In this lesson you will explore various cultural differences and how nursing care should be adapted to meet each patient's individual needs. Begin this activity by reviewing the general concepts presented in your textbook. Answer the following questions to solidify your understanding of culture.

/ **Clinical Preparation: Writing Activity**

⏱ 10 minutes

1. Define *cultural competence.*

2. Using the definitions of culture provided in the textbook, describe culture in your own words.

3. The three major methods for assessing the culture of a client are _____,

_____, and _____.

 ### CD-ROM Activity

45 minutes

- Sign in to work at Pacific View Regional Hospital for Period of Care 1. (*Note:* If you are already in the virtual hospital from a previous exercise, click on **Leave the Floor** and then **Restart the Program** to get to the sign-in window.)
- From the Patient List, select Piya Jordan (Room 403), Clarence Hughes (Room 404), and Pablo Rodriguez (Room 405).
- Click on **Go to Nurses' Station**.
- Click on **Chart** and then on **403** for Piya Jordan's chart.
- Click on **History and Physical**.

1. Read Piya Jordan's H&P and document her cultural needs and/or considerations below. Complete the table by repeating the above steps for Clarence Hughes and Pablo Rodriguez.

Patient	Cultural Needs/Considerations
Piya Jordan (Room 403)	
Clarence Hughes (Room 404)	
Pablo Rodriguez (Room 405)	

→ • Click on **Return to Nurses' Station**.
  • Click on **403** on the bottom tool bar to enter Piya Jordan's room.
  • Read the Initial Observation.
  • Click on **Patient Care** and then **Nurse-Client Interactions**.
  • Select and view the video titled **0735: Pain-Adverse Drug Event**. (*Note:* Check the virtual clock to see whether enough time has elapsed. You can use the fast-forward feature to advance the time by 2-minute intervals if the video is not yet available. Then click again on **Patient Care** and **Nurse-Client Interactions** to refresh the screen.)

 2. Based on this video, what culturally sensitive concepts (see textbook pages 59-61) should be identified and/or explored when planning care for Piya Jordan?

→ • Now click on **404** at the bottom of your screen to enter Clarence Hughes' room.
  • Read the Initial Observation.
  • Click on **Patient Care** and then **Nurse-Client Interactions**.
  • Click on and view the video titled **0730: Assessment/Perception of Care**.

 3. Based on this video, what culturally sensitive concepts (see textbook pages 59-61) can the nurse identify that are relevant for Clarence Hughes?

→ • Click on **405** at bottom of screen to enter Pablo Rodriguez's room.
  • Read the Initial Observation.
  • Click on **Patient Care** and then **Nurse-Client Interactions**.
  • Click on and view the video titled **0730: Symptom Management**.

4. Describe how Pablo Rodriguez's comments reveal his cultural beliefs.

5. Using the nursing process, develop a culturally sensitive nursing care plan for Clarence Hughes related to the two client problems identified in the first column of the table below: (1) pain and (2) spiritual/cultural needs. Document your plan in the remaining columns.

Patient Problems (Assessment)	Nursing Diagnosis	Goals/ Outcomes (Planning)	Nursing Interventions	Evaluation
Pain				
Spiritual/ cultural needs				

LESSON 2 _____

Pain

👓 **Reading Assignment:** Pain: The Fifth Vital Sign (Chapter 7)

Patients: Clarence Hughes, Room 404
Pablo Rodriguez, Room 405

Goal: Demonstrate understanding and appropriate application of pain management concepts.

Objectives:

1. Define the concept of *pain.*
2. Describe the source and type of pain for each patient.
3. Perform a comprehensive pain assessment for each patient.
4. Identify variables that influence each patient's perception of pain.
5. Safely administer analgesic medications to a patient experiencing pain.
6. Plan appropriate nonpharmacologic measures that may be used to treat each patient's pain.

In this lesson you will evaluate the pain experience of two different patients—from assessment to management. Clarence Hughes is a 73-year-old male who is status post total knee arthroplasty. Pablo Rodriguez is a 71-year-old male admitted with advanced non-small-cell lung carcinoma. Begin this activity by reviewing the general concepts presented in your textbook. Answer the following questions to solidify your understanding of pain.

✒️ **Clinical Preparation: Writing Activity**

 10 minutes

1. Using the three definitions of pain provided in the textbook, describe pain in your own words.

CD-ROM Activity

45 minutes

Exercise 1

- Sign in to work at Pacific View Regional Hospital for Period of Care 1. (*Note:* If you are already in the virtual hospital from a previous exercise, click on **Leave the Floor** and then **Restart the Program** to get to the sign-in window.)
- From the Patient List, select Clarence Hughes (Room 404) and click on **Get Report**.

1. What data are provided in the report concerning this client's most recent pain assessment?

Now complete your own pain assessment on Clarence Hughes.

 • Click on **Go to Nurses' Station**.
- Click on Room **404**; then select **Take Vital Signs** (just above Initial Observations).

2. How does Clarence Hughes rate his pain at the present time?

 • Click on **Patient Care** and then **Physical Assessment**.

3. Perform a focused assessment on Clarence Hughes. Document your findings below.

 • Click on **Patient Care** and then **Nurse-Client Interactions**.
- Select and view the video titled **0730: Assessment/Perception of Care**. (*Note:* Check the virtual clock to see whether enough time has elapsed. You can use the fast-forward feature to advance the time by 2-minute intervals if the video is not yet available. Then click again on **Patient Care** and **Nurse-Client Interactions** to refresh the screen.)

4. How does Clarence Hughes describe his pain? Describe his nonverbal communication. Do his nonverbal cues correlate with his complaint of pain?

5. The nurse asks Clarence Hughes whether she may perform an assessment before medicating him for pain. Is this appropriate? Why or why not?

→ • Click on **EPR** near the upper right corner of your screen.
  • Your name and password should appear automatically; click on **Login**.
  • Click on the down arrow next to the Patient field. From the drop-down menu, select **404**.
  • Select **Vital Signs** as the category.

6. Document Clarence Hughes' pain rating and characteristics over the last 24 hours in the table provided below. (*Note:* You will complete the table in question 7.)

→ • Click on **Exit EPR**.
  • Click on **Chart** and then on **404** for Clarence Hughes' chart.
  • Within the chart, click on the **Expired MARs** tab.

7. Review the expired MARs for Clarence Hughes, noting the times of analgesic administration. Document your findings in the far right column in the table below.

Time of Assessment	Pain Rating	Pain Characteristic	Name of Analgesic Administered
Tuesday 0700			
Tuesday 0815			
Tuesday 0930			
Tuesday 1230			
Tuesday 1330			
Tuesday 1500			
Tuesday 1630			
Tuesday 1700			
Tuesday 2030			
Tuesday 2300			
Wednesday 0200			
Wednesday 0715			

➤ • Click on **Return to Room 404**.
  • Click on **Kardex**.
  • Click on tab **404** for Clarence Hughes' records.

8. What is the stated outcome related to comfort for Clarence Hughes? Is this a measurable outcome? How might you improve on the writing of the outcome?

9. Based on the stated outcome, review the table you completed in questions 6 and 7. Was the pain medication administered effective? Give a rationale for your answer.

10. Was the client's pain assessed appropriately following each analgesic administration? Explain your answer.

11. What is the physiologic source of Clarence Hughes' pain? What type of pain is he experiencing? Explain your answer. (*Hint:* See pages 64 and 74 of your textbook.)

12. Is the ordered analgesic medication appropriate for this type of pain? If not, what would you suggest? Are there any nonpharmacologic interventions that might be helpful for Clarence Hughes? Explain your answer.

13. What nursing assessment should be completed prior to administration of oxycodone with acetaminophen?

14. What common side effects should the nurse monitor for related to opioid use? (*Hint:* If you need help, return to the Nurses' Station and click on the **Drug Guide** on the counter.)

→ • Click on **Return to Room 404**.
  • Click on **Chart.**
  • Click on **404** for Clarence Hughes' chart.
  • Click on the **Nurse's Notes** tab and review the notes.

15. According to the note for Wednesday at 0715, which of the side effects (identified in question 14) is Clarence Hughes experiencing? What should the nurse do to treat and/or prevent this side effect?

Since Clarence Hughes received his last dose of pain medication at 0200, it is now appropriate to administer another dose. Prepare to administer a dose of analgesic to him by completing the following steps:

→ • Click **Medication Room** on the bottom of your screen.
  • Access the **Automated System** by either selecting that icon at the top of screen or clicking on the Automated System cart in center of screen.
  • Click on **Login**.
  • Choose Clarence Hughes in box 1 and Automated System Drawer (G-O) in box 2. Click **Open Drawer** and review the list of available medications. (*Note:* You may click **Review MAR** at any time to verify correct medication order. Remember to look at patient name on MAR to make sure you have the correct MAR—you must click on the correct room number within the MAR. Click on **Return to Medication Room** after reviewing the correct MAR.)
  • From the Open Drawer view, select the correct medication to administer. Click **Put Medication on Tray** and then on **Close Drawer**.
  • Click on **View Medication Room**.
  • Begin the preparation process by clicking on **Preparation** at the top of screen or clicking on the tray on the counter on the left side of the Medication Room.
  • Click **Prepare**, fill in any requested data in the Preparation Wizard, and click **Next**. Then select the correct patient and click **Finish**.
  • You can click on **Review Your Medications** and then on **Return to Medication Room** when ready. Once you are back in the Medication Room, you may go directly to Clarence Hughes' room to administer this medication by clicking on **404** at the bottom of the screen.
  • Administer the medication, utilizing the five rights of medication administration. After you have collected the appropriate assessment data and are ready for administration, click **Patient Care** and then **Medication Administration**. Verify that the correct patient and medication(s) appear in the left-hand window. Then click the down arrow next to Select. From the drop-down menu, select **Administer** and complete the Administration Wizard by providing any information requested. When the Wizard stops asking for information, click **Administer to Patient**. Specify **Yes** when asked whether this administration should be recorded in the MAR. Finally, click **Finish**.

Now let's see how you did!

→ • Click on **Leave the Floor** at the bottom of your screen. From the Floor Menu, select **Look at Your Preceptor's Evaluation**. Then click on **Medication Scorecard**.

16. Disregard the report for the routine scheduled medications but note below whether or not you correctly administered the analgesic medication. If not, why do you think you were incorrect in administering this drug? According to Table C in this scorecard, what are the appropriate resources that should be used prior to administering this medication? Did you utilize them correctly?

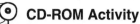 **CD-ROM Activity**

45 minutes

Exercise 2

- Sign in to work at Pacific View Regional Hospital for Period of Care 1. (*Note:* If you are already in the virtual hospital from a previous exercise, click on **Leave the Floor** and then **Restart the Program** to get to the sign-in window.)
- From the Patient List, select Pablo Rodriguez (Room 405) and click on **Get Report**.

1. What information is provided in the report concerning Pablo Rodriguez's most recent pain assessment?

Now let's complete your own pain assessment on Pablo Rodriguez.

- Click on **Go to Nurses' Station**.
- Click on **405**.
- Click on **Take Vital Signs**.

2. How does Pablo Rodriguez rate his pain at the present time?

- Click on **Patient Care** and then **Physical Assessment**.

3. Perform a focused assessment on Pablo Rodriguez. Document your findings below.

• Click on **Chart**.
  • Click on **405** for Pablo Rodriguez's chart.
  • Click on **Nursing Admission**.

4. Scroll down to page 22 of the Nursing Admission form. What are the aggravating and alleviating factors related to Pablo Rodriguez's pain?

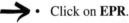 • Click on **Return to Room 405**.
  • Click on **Patient Care** and then **Nurse-Client Interactions**.
  • Click on video titled **0730: Symptom Management**. (*Note:* Check the virtual clock to see whether enough time has elapsed. You can use the fast-forward feature to advance the time by 2-minute intervals if the video is not yet available. Then click again on **Patient Care** and **Nurse-Client Interactions** to refresh the screen.)

5. What cultural influences are affecting this client's perception and management of pain?

  • Click on **EPR**.
  • Click on **Login**.
  • Select **405** from the drop-down menu next to Patient.
  • Choose **Vital Signs** as the category.

6. In the table on the next page, document Pablo Rodriguez's pain rating and characteristics since admission. (*Note:* You will complete this table in question 7.)

  • Now click on **Exit EPR**.
  • Click on **Chart**.
  • Select **405**.
  • Click on **Expired MARs**.

7. Review the expired MARs, noting the times of analgesic administration. Document your findings in the table on the next page.

Time of Assessment	Pain Rating	Pain Characteristic	Time of Medication Administration	Name of Analgesic Administered
Tuesday 2300				
			Wednesday 0100	
Wednesday 0300				
Wednesday 0700			Wednesday 0700	

- Click on **Return to Room 405**.
- Click on **Kardex**.
- Click on tab **405** for Pablo Rodriguez's records.

8. What is the stated outcome related to comfort for Pablo Rodriguez? Is this a measurable outcome? How might you improve on the writing of the outcome?

9. Based on the stated outcome, review the table you completed in questions 6 and 7, as well as your pain assessment in question 2. Was the pain medication administered effective? Give a rationale for your answer.

10. Was the client's pain assessed appropriately following each analgesic administration? Explain your answer.

11. What is the physiologic source of Pablo Rodriguez's pain? What type of pain is he experiencing? Explain your answer. (*Hint:* See pages 64 and 74 of your textbook.)

12. Is the ordered analgesic medication appropriate for this type of pain? If not, what would you suggest? Are there any nonpharmacologic interventions that might be helpful for Pablo Rodriguez? Explain your answer.

- Click on **Return to Room 405**.
- Click on **Patient Care** and then **Nurse-Client Interactions**.
- Click on video titled **0735: Patient Perceptions**. (*Note:* Check the virtual clock to see whether enough time has elapsed. You can use the fast-forward feature to advance the time by 2-minute intervals if the video is not yet available. Then click again on **Patient Care** and **Nurse-Client Interactions** to refresh the screen.)

13. Discuss the nurse's evaluation of Pablo Rodriguez's understanding and use of the PCA pump. Do you think the nurse's actions are therapeutic? If not, what other approaches would you suggest?

14. What nursing assessments and interventions are appropriate for clients receiving IV morphine sulfate? (*Hint:* For help, click on the **Drug** icon in the lower left corner of the screen.)

Substance Abuse

Reading Assignment: Substance Abuse (Chapter 8)

Patient: Harry George, Room 401

Goal: Demonstrate understanding and appropriate application of health care concepts related to substance abuse.

Objectives:

1. Identify risk factors associated with substance abuse.
2. Describe assessment findings related to the use of nicotine and alcohol.
3. Describe assessment findings related to withdrawal from nicotine and alcohol.
4. Examine alcohol withdrawal protocols for the care of a patient admitted to an acute care setting.
5. Identify appropriate nursing interventions when caring for a patient with substance abuse.

In this lesson you will learn about the care of a patient undergoing specific substance abuse issues. Harry George is a 54-year-old male admitted with infection and swelling of his left foot and a history of type 2 diabetes. Begin this activity by reviewing the general concepts presented in your textbook. Answer the following questions to solidify your understanding of substance abuse.

Clinical Preparation: Writing Activity

10 minutes

1. Define *substance abuse*.

57

2. Define *dependence.*

3. List three criteria that must be present to document a nursing diagnosis of substance abuse.

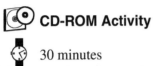 **CD-ROM Activity**

30 minutes

Exercise 1

- Sign in to work at Pacific View Regional Hospital for Period of Care 1. (*Note:* If you are already in the virtual hospital from a previous exercise, click on **Leave the Floor** and then **Restart the Program** to get to the sign-in window.)
- From the Patient List, select Harry George (Room 401).
- Click on **Go to Nurses' Station**.
- Click on **Chart** at top of the screen or on the rack of charts in the center of the screen.
- Click on **401** to view Harry George's chart.
- Click on the **Emergency Department** tab and review this record.

1. What are Harry George's primary and secondary diagnoses?

2. What specific risk factors for alcoholism are noted in the Emergency Department Record? (*Hint:* Read the admitting physician's notes.) Describe how the risk factors contribute to alcohol abuse.

3. Although unknown for this client, what other potential risk factors for alcoholism could be contributing to Harry George's substance abuse? (*Hint:* See pages 92-93 of textbook.)

4. When did Harry George begin drinking excessively? Was there a precipitating event that contributed to this problem?

5. What other documentation is found in the Emergency Department notes to support the diagnosis of alcohol abuse?

6. Is there any evidence of nicotine addiction?

→ • Still within the chart, click on the **History and Physical** tab.

7. Read the physical examination report on page 4 of the H&P. What assessment findings may be related to Harry George's alcohol abuse?

8. What further history can you find regarding nicotine abuse?

9. What physical examination finding may be related to cigarette smoking?

 • Now click on **Laboratory Reports**.

10. What is Harry George's blood alcohol level?

11. What clinical manifestations would you expect to find based on this level? (*Hint:* See page 100 of your textbook.)

 • Click on **Return to Nurses' Station** at the bottom of your screen.
   • Click on **401** to go to Harry George's room.
   • Click on **Patient Care** and then **Nurse-Client Interactions**.
   • Click on the video titled **0735: Symptom Management**. (*Note:* Check the virtual clock to see whether enough time has elapsed. You can use the fast-forward feature to advance the time by 2-minute intervals if the video is not yet available. Then click again on **Patient Care** and **Nurse-Client Interactions** to refresh the screen.)

12. What visual assessment findings noted in this video might suggest withdrawal symptoms for Harry George?

CD-ROM Activity

45 minutes

Exercise 2

- Sign in to work at Pacific View Regional Hospital for Period of Care 4. (*Note:* If you are already in the virtual hospital from a previous exercise, click on **Leave the Floor** and then **Restart the Program** to get to the sign-in window.)
- Click on **Chart** and then on **401** for Harry George's chart. (*Remember:* You are not able to visit patients or administer medications during Period of Care 4. You are able to review patients' records only.)
- Click on the **Mental Health** tab.

1. Read the Psychiatric/Mental Health Assessment for Harry George. What risk factors for substance abuse are noted on this assessment?

- Click on **Nurse's Notes**.

2. How does the nurse describe Harry George's behavior now?

3. The textbook identifies the following symptoms of clients experiencing alcohol withdrawal. Put an X next to each symptom that applies to Harry George.

_____ Tremors

_____ Jerking movements

_____ Vomiting

_____ Diaphoresis, tenting skin

_____ Undernourished

_____ Dehydrated

_____ Increased pulse and blood pressure

_____ Disoriented to place, time

_____ No appetite

_____ Reports "shaking inside"

_____ Nausea

_____ Delusional

_____ Hallucinating

4. Symptoms of withdrawal can be categorized as minor, major, or life-threatening. How would you classify Harry George's symptoms? (*Hint:* See page 100 of textbook.)

 • Click on **History and Physical**.

5. At the end of the History and Physical, the physician writes a plan of care. What pharmacologic interventions is the physician planning to prevent and/or treat alcohol withdrawal?

6. What is the intended benefit of thiamine administration for this client? (*Hint:* You may consult the Drug Guide located in the Nurses' Station.)

7. What is the classification of the drug chlordiazepoxide and what is its most common brand name? What is the intended therapeutic effect of this drug for Harry George?

 • Still in the chart, click on **Nurse's Notes**.

8. Read the notes dated Wednesday at 1245 and at 1315. Is the chlordiazepoxide effective? Explain.

9. What is the classification of lorazepam and what is its most common brand name? What is the intended therapeutic effect of this drug for Harry George?

10. Are there any potential drug interactions between chlordiazepoxide and lorazepam? If so, please describe.

11. Since both Librium and Ativan are ordered for similar therapeutic effects, what factors would influence the nurse's decision regarding which of these medications to use. (*Hint:* Consult the MAR.)

→ • Click on **Physician's Orders**.

12. What is the most recent physician order?

→ • Click on **Physician's Notes**.

13. Read the most recent physician's progress note. What is the rationale for writing the order you identified in question 12?

14. Based on your readings in the textbook (see page 101), what interventions would you expect to be part of an Alcohol Withdrawal Protocol?

→ • Once again, click on **Nurse's Notes**.

15. Read the note for Wednesday at 1800. What clinical manifestations of nicotine withdrawal is the client exhibiting?

16. According to your textbook, after how many hours of abstinence do nicotine withdrawal symptoms begin to appear?

17. How long has Harry George been without cigarettes? (*Hint:* Look at time and date of the first Nurse's Note.)

18. What is the effect of simultaneous alcohol and nicotine withdrawal?

19. What typical manifestations of nicotine withdrawal might be found in another client withdrawing *only* from nicotine?

20. To plan nursing care for Harry George, identify three priority nursing diagnoses for the client problems identified in the table below. For each diagnosis, identify related client outcomes and appropriate nursing interventions to achieve these outcomes.

Patient Problems (Assessment)	Nursing Diagnosis	Goals/Outcomes (Planning)	Nursing Interventions
Tremors			
Anxiety			
Malnutrition			

LESSON 4

End-of-Life Care

 Reading Assignment: End-of-Life Care (Chapter 9)

Patient: Pablo Rodriguez, Room 405

Goal: Demonstrate understanding and appropriate application of end-of-life concepts related to health care.

Objectives:

1. Identify appropriate application of palliative care concepts for a patient with a terminal illness.
2. Assess and identify common symptoms of distress present in a terminally ill patient.
3. Choose interventions appropriate to relieve symptoms of distress in a terminally ill patient.
4. Describe appropriate communication techniques when dealing with a terminally ill patient and family.

In this lesson you will describe, plan, and evaluate the care of a patient with a terminal illness that is no longer responding to therapy. Pablo Rodriguez is a 71-year-old male suffering from advanced non-small-cell lung carcinoma diagnosed 1 year ago.

CD-ROM Activity

30 minutes

Exercise 1

- Sign in to work at Pacific View Regional Hospital for Period of Care 3. (*Note:* If you are already in the virtual hospital from a previous exercise, click on **Leave the Floor** and then **Restart the Program** to get to the sign-in window.)
- From the Patient List, select Pablo Rodriguez (Room 405).
- Click on **Go to Nurses' Station**.
- Click on **Chart** and then on **405**.
- Click on the **Emergency Department** tab and review this record.

1. Why was Pablo Rodriguez admitted to the hospital?

2. What are Pablo Rodriguez's primary and secondary diagnoses?

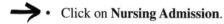

 • Click on **Nursing Admission**.

3. What does the admitting nurse document as this client's anticipated needs for support at the time of discharge?

4. Does the client have a signed advance directive?

 5. What does the Patient Self-Determination Act of 1990 require health care agencies to provide to clients without an advance directive? (*Hint:* See textbook page 106.)

 • Click on **Nurse's Notes**.

6. Based on available documentation, do you think the admitting nurse complied with the Patient Self-Determination Act of 1990? Explain.

 • Click on **Return to Nurses' Station**.
• Click on **Kardex**.
• Click on tab **405**.

7. What is Pablo Rodriguez's code status? Is this appropriate based on the reason for this admission? (*Hint:* See your answer for question 1.) Explain.

→ • Click on **Return to Nurses' Station**.

- Click on **405** at the bottom of your screen.

- Select **Patient Care** and then **Nurse-Client Interactions**.

- Select the video titled **1530: Decision—End-of-Life Care**. (*Note:* Check the virtual clock to see whether enough time has elapsed. You can use the fast-forward feature to advance the time by 2-minute intervals if the video is not yet available. Then click again on **Patient Care** and **Nurse-Client Interactions** to refresh the screen.)

8. What is Pablo Rodriguez telling the nurse?

9. What therapeutic communication techniques is the nurse using? Are they effective? What other technique(s) might have been used?

 10. What would you do if Pablo Rodriguez asked you to administer a lethal dose of morphine to "stop my pain and help me die with dignity"? What legal term would apply to this request? (*Hint:* See page 116 of textbook.)

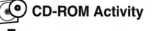 **CD-ROM Activity**

45 minutes

Exercise 2

- Sign in to work at Pacific View Regional Hospital for Period of Care 1. (*Note:* If you are already in the virtual hospital from a previous exercise, click on **Leave the Floor** and then **Restart the Program** to get to the sign-in window.)
- From the Patient List, select Pablo Rodriguez (Room 405).
- Click on **Go to Nurses' Station**.
- Click on **405** to go to the patient's room.

1. According to the Initial Observation report on Pablo Rodriguez, what physical symptom of distress is he displaying?

2. Identify interventions you would use to alleviate Pablo Rodriguez's symptoms. Provide rationales for your interventions. (*Hint:* You may need to go to the client's chart to review physician orders and/or use the Drug Guide to provide rationales.)

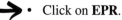 - Click on **EPR**.
- Click **Login**.
- Select **405** from the drop-down menu next to Patient box.
- With **Vital Signs** as the selected category, find the vital sign assessment documented at 0700. (*Hint:* Use the backward and forward arrows to scroll between times.)

3. Describe Pablo Rodriguez's pain assessment.

4. What interventions would be appropriate to relieve this pain?

Now let's check the client's current vital signs.

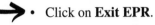 • Click on **Exit EPR**.
- Click on **Take Vital Signs**. (Note that pain assessment is now considered the fifth vital sign.)

5. Based on the EPR data and Pablo Rodriguez's current pain rating, is the morphine providing effective relief? Explain.

- Click on **Patient Care** and then **Physical Assessment**.
 • From the list of body areas, click on **Abdomen**.
- From the system subcategories, click on **Gastrointestinal**.

6. Document your assessment findings below. What is this significance of these findings? How do they relate to Pablo Rodriguez's diagnosis and/or treatment?

7. How would you intervene to prevent potential complications related to the above findings?

- Click on **Patient Care** and then **Nurse-Client Interactions**.
 • Select and view the video titled **0730: Symptom Management**. (*Note:* Check the virtual clock to see whether enough time has elapsed. You can use the fast-forward feature to advance the time by 2-minute intervals if the video is not yet available. Then click again on **Patient Care** and **Nurse-Client Interactions** to refresh the screen.)

8. Describe Pablo Rodriguez's emotional distress as displayed in this video.

9. What nursing interventions would be appropriate to help Pablo Rodriguez cope?

➡ • Select and view the video titled **0735: Patient Perceptions**. (*Note:* Check the virtual clock to see whether enough time has elapsed. You can use the fast-forward feature to advance the time by 2-minute intervals if the video is not yet available. Then click again on **Patient Care** and **Nurse-Client Interactions** to refresh the screen.)

10. Now that his pain has been controlled, what two physical symptoms of distress does Pablo Rodriguez complain of? For each of his symptoms, identify interventions you could use to relieve these discomforts.

11. Recall the goals for end-of-life care as described in your textbook. Are these being met for Pablo Rodriguez? Explain.

LESSON 5 _____

Fluid Imbalance

_____

Reading Assignment: Fluid and Electrolyte Balance (Chapter 14)
                          Interventions for Clients with Fluid Imbalances (Chapter 15)

Patients: Piya Jordan, Room 403
                Patricia Newman, Room 406

Goal: Utilize the nursing process to competently care for patients with fluid, electrolyte,
            and/or acid-base imbalances.

Objectives:

1. Identify normal physiologic influences on fluid and electrolyte balance.
2. Compare and contrast the pathophysiology related to dehydration and overhydration.
3. Utilize laboratory data and clinical manifestations to assess fluid balance and imbalance.
4. Describe collaborative management strategies used to maintain and/or restore fluid balance.
5. Critically analyze differences in fluid balance assessment findings between two patients.
6. Develop an appropriate plan of care for patients displaying fluid imbalances.

In this lesson you will assess, plan, and implement care for two patients with similar but differing fluid imbalances. Piya Jordan is a 68-year-old female admitted with nausea and vomiting for several days following weeks of poor appetite and increasing weakness. Patricia Newman is a 61-year-old female admitted with dyspnea at rest, cough, and fever. You will begin this lesson by reviewing the general concepts of fluid homeostasis as presented in your textbook. Answer the following questions to cement your understanding of the normal physiologic concepts related to fluid balance.

Clinical Preparation: Writing Activity

30 minutes

1. Describe the functions of body water.

2. Identify the two fluid compartments in the body and describe their composition.

3. Compare and contrast the pathophysiologic basis of the three types of dehydration and over-hydration by completing the table below.

Dehydration Disorder	Pathophysiology	Overhydration Disorder	Pathophysiology
Isotonic dehydration		Isotonic overhydration	
Hypotonic dehydration		Hypotonic overhydration	
Hypertonic dehydration		Hypertonic overhydration	

4. Match each of the following terms related to fluid volume regulation with its corresponding definition.

Term

_____ Hydrostatic pressure

_____ Colloidal oncotic pressure

_____ Filtration

_____ Albumin

_____ Diffusion

_____ Osmolarity

_____ Aldosterone

_____ Hypotonic

_____ Osmosis

_____ Antidiuretic hormone

_____ Isotonic

_____ Permeable membrane

_____ Solute

_____ Facilitated diffusion

_____ Hypertonic

_____ Active transport

Definition

a. Passive transport of a solute across a membrane

b. The movement of fluid through a cell or blood vessel membrane because of hydrostatic pressure differences on the two sides of the membrane

c. Movement of water only from an area of higher water concentration to an area of lower water concentration

d. The force of pressure exerted by static water in a confined space—"water-pushing" pressure

e. Separates two fluid compartments and permits the movement of one or more substances (by diffusion) from one compartment to the other

f. The concentration of particles in 1000 mL of water

g. The solid particle dissolved in a solution

h. Any solution with a solute concentration equal to the osmolarity of normal body fluids or normal saline, about 300 mOsm/L

i. A hormone produced by the hypothalamus and released by the posterior pituitary gland to regulate body water

j. Assisted movement of a substance through a permeable membrane between two fluid compartments; occurs down a concentration gradient

k. A common protein in the plasma that is responsible for pulling or absorbing fluid from the interstitial spaces

l. A hormone produced by the adrenal cortex that affects the kidneys' resorption of sodium and water in the renal tubules

m. Assisted movement of a substance through a permeable membrane between two fluid compartments; requires the expenditure of chemical energy

n. Any solution with a solute concentration (osmolarity) greater than that of normal body fluids (>310 mOsm/L)

o. The osmotic pressure exerted by the concentration of proteins within a solution—pulls fluid back into the blood vessel from the interstitial space

p. Any solution with a solute concentration (osmolarity) less than that of normal body fluids (<270 mOsm/L)

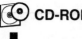 **CD-ROM Activity**

 30 minutes

Exercise 1

- Sign in to work at Pacific View Regional Hospital for Period of Care 1. (*Note:* If you are already in the virtual hospital from a previous exercise, click on **Leave the Floor** and then **Restart the Program** to get to the sign-in window.)
- From the Patient List, select Piya Jordan (Room 403).
- Click on **Go to Nurses' Station**.
- Click on **Chart** and then on **403**.
- Click on **Emergency Department** and review this record.

1. Record findings below that support the diagnosis of dehydration.

 • Click on **Nursing Admission**.

2. Are there any additional findings noted on this document that support the diagnosis of dehydration? If so, list them below.

• Click on **Laboratory Reports**.

3. Record pertinent results below and describe the significance of each result in relation to the diagnosis of dehydration.

4. Based on the above findings, what type of dehydration do you think Piya Jordan is suffering from?

→ • Click on **History and Physical.**

    5. Based on your review of Piya Jordan's History and Physical, what were the contributing factors leading to her dehydration?

→ • Click on **Physician's Orders**.

    6. Identify orders that are appropriate management strategies for the treatment of dehydration and write your findings below.

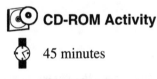

CD-ROM Activity

45 minutes

Exercise 2

Now you will answer similar questions related to fluid balance for another client and compare your findings.

- Sign in to work at Pacific View Regional Hospital for Period of Care 1. (*Note:* If you are already in the virtual hospital from a previous exercise, click on **Leave the Floor** and then **Restart the Program** to get to the sign-in window.)
- From the Patient List, select Patricia Newman (Room 406).
- Click on **Go to Nurses' Station**.
- Click on **Chart** and then on **406**.
- Click on **Emergency Department** and review this record.

    1. Identify assessment findings related to fluid balance and record them below. How do these findings differ from those for Piya Jordan? Are there any similarities?

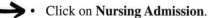 • Click on **Nursing Admission**.

2. Are there any additional findings noted on this document related to fluid balance and/or imbalance? If so, list them below. How do they compare with findings for Piya Jordan?

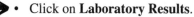 • Click on **Laboratory Results**.

3. Record pertinent results below and describe the significance of each result in relation to fluid balance. Describe any differences between these findings and those for Piya Jordan.

4. Based on your findings, does Patricia Newman have a fluid imbalance? If so, what type?

5. What are the contributing factors for this client's potential or actual fluid imbalance?

➤ • Click on **History and Physical**.

6. What coexisting illness might have an impact on the selection and rate of IV fluid therapy?

7. Develop an appropriate plan of care for clients with either dehydration or overhydration by completing the table below.

Collaborative Plan of Care	Dehydration	Overhydration
Client outcomes		
Assessment parameters		
Diet therapy		
Drug therapy		

Electrolyte Imbalances, Part 1

/O尺O **Reading Assignment:** Fluid and Electrolyte Balance (Chapter 14)
Interventions for Clients with Electrolyte Imbalances
(Chapter 16)

Patients: Piya Jordan, Room 403
Patricia Newman, Room 406

Goal: Utilize the nursing process to competently care for patients with electrolyte imbalances.

Objectives:

1. Describe normal physiologic influences on electrolyte balance.
2. Identify specific etiologic factors related to hypokalemia for assigned patients.
3. Research potential drug interactions related to hypokalemia for assigned patients.
4. Assess patients for clinical manifestations related to hypo- and hyperkalemia.
5. Utilize the nursing process to correctly administer IV potassium chloride per physician orders.

In this lesson you will assess, plan, and implement care for two patients with hypokalemia. Piya Jordan is a 68-year-old female admitted with nausea and vomiting for several days following weeks of poor appetite and increasing weakness. Patricia Newman is a 61-year-old female admitted with pneumonia and a 12-year history of emphysema. You will begin this lesson by reviewing the general functions of electrolytes within the body as presented in your textbook. Answer the following questions to cement your understanding of the normal physiologic concepts related to potassium balance.

✎ **Clinical Preparation: Writing Activity**

🕐 15 minutes

1. Describe the general functions of electrolytes within the body.

2. Define the following terms:

   a. Ion

   b. Cation

   c. Anion

3. Identify the specific functions of potassium within the body.

4. Describe the physiologic influences on potassium balance.

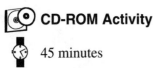 **CD-ROM Activity**

45 minutes

Exercise 1

- Sign in to work at Pacific View Regional Hospital for Period of Care 1. (*Note:* If you are already in the virtual hospital from a previous exercise, click on **Leave the Floor** and then **Restart the Program** to get to the sign-in window.)
- From the Patient List, select Piya Jordan (Room 403).
- Click on **Go to Nurses' Station.**
- Click on **Chart** and then on **403**.
- Click on **Laboratory Reports**.

1. What was Piya Jordan's initial potassium level on Monday at 2200?

 • Click on **Emergency Department** and review this record.

2. What would be the most likely cause for hypokalemia in this client?

3. What did the physician order to treat this electrolyte imbalance? Is this appropriate? Is the dilution and rate safe to administer?

 • Click again on **Laboratory Reports**.

4. What was Piya Jordan's potassium level for Tuesday at 0630? Was the physician's order for potassium effective? Is there any cause for concern?

 • Click on **Return to Nurses' Station**.
 • Click on **403** at the bottom of your screen to go to Piya Jordan's room.
 • Click on **Patient Care** and then **Physical Assessment**.

5. Complete a physical assessment on Piya Jordan, specifically looking for clinical manifestations of hypokalemia. (*Hint:* Refer to textbook pages 227-228.) Document your findings in the table below and underline or highlight those that correlate with hypokalemia.

Areas Assessed	Findings on Physical Examination
Cardiovascular	
Respiratory	
Neuromuscular	
Gastrointestinal	
Renal	

6. What was the potassium level that was drawn on Wednesday at 0630?

7. Explain the etiology for this recurrence of hypokalemia.

- Click on **Chart** at the top of your screen.
- Click on **403** for Piya Jordan's chart.
- Click on **Physician's Orders**.

8. What did the physician order in response to today's potassium level?

Prepare to administer this ordered dose of potassium chloride to Piya Jordan by completing the following steps.

- Click on **Return to Room 403**.
- Click **Medication Room** on the bottom of your screen.
- Click on **IV Storage** near the top of your screen (*Note:* You can also click on any of the three bins just above the refrigerator.) Either of these methods will bring up a close-up view of the IV storage bins.
- Click on the bin labeled **Small Volume** and review the list of available medications. (*Note:* You may click on **Review MAR** at any time to verify correct medication order. Remember to look at the patient name on the MAR to make sure you have the correct patient's record—you must click on the correct room number within the MAR. Click on **Return to Medication Room** after reviewing the correct MAR.)
- From the list of medications in the bin, select **potassium chloride**. Then click **Put Medication on Tray** and **Close Bin**.
- Click **View Medication Room**.
- Click on **Preparation** at the top of the screen or on the preparation tray on the counter. Select the correct medication to administer; then click **Prepare**.
- Wait for instructions or questions from the Preparation Wizard. Then click **Next**.
- Choose the correct patient to administer this medication to. Click **Finish**.
- You can click **Review Your Medications** and then **Return to Medication Room** when ready. From the Medication Room, go directly to Piya Jordan's room by clicking on **403** at bottom of screen.

Prior to administering intravenous medications, the patient's IV site must be assessed.

- Click on **Patient Care** and then **Physical Assessment**.
- Click on **Upper Extremities**.
- Select **Integumentary** from the system subcategories.

9. Document the IV site assessment findings below. Is it appropriate to administer the IV potassium at this time? What other steps should you take to ensure you have adequately addressed the five rights of medication administration?

➤ • After you have collected the appropriate assessment data and are ready for administration, click on **Medication Administration**. (*Note:* If you are not still in the Patient Care screen, you will need to first click **Patient Care** and then choose **Medication Administration**.)

• To the right of the medication name, next to Select, click the down arrow and choose **Administer** from the drop-down menu.

• Complete the Administration Wizard and click **Administer to Patient** when done.

• Check **Yes** when asked whether this drug administration should be documented on the MAR.

• Now click on **MAR** at the top of your screen.

10. What are Piya Jordan's scheduled AM medications? What medication would you question giving her, and for what reason?

11. Piya Jordan complains of pain at the IV site while the potassium is infusing. What interventions might be used at this point?

Now let's see how you did!

➤ • Click on **Leave the Floor** at the bottom of your screen. From the Floor Menu, select **Look at Your Preceptor's Evaluation**. Then click on **Medication Scorecard**.

12. Disregard the report for the routine scheduled medications, but note below whether or not you correctly administered the potassium chloride. If not, why do you think you were incorrect in administering this drug? According to Table C in this scorecard, what are the appropriate resources that should be used and important assessments that should be completed prior to administering this medication? Did you utilize and perform them correctly?

CD-ROM Activity

30 minutes

Exercise 2

- Sign in to work at Pacific View Regional Hospital for Period of Care 1. (*Note:* If you are still in the virtual hospital from Exercise 1, click on **Leave the Floor** and then **Restart the Program** to get to the sign-in window.)
- From the Patient List, select Patricia Newman (Room 406).
- Click on **Go to Nurses' Station**.
- Click on **Chart** and then on **406**.
- Click on **Laboratory Reports**.

1. What was Patricia Newman's initial potassium level this morning?

- Click on **History and Physical**.

2. What would be the most likely cause for hypokalemia in this client?

- Click on **Physician's Orders**.

3. What did the physician order to treat this electrolyte imbalance?

4. What is missing from this order?

5. Where could you verify this missing information?

6. What is the difference between the treatment of hypokalemia for Piya Jordan and that for Patricia Newman? Provide a rationale for the difference.

7. Look again at the physician's orders. Is there an order for any follow-up lab work?

8. What is the nurse's responsibility in regard to follow-up lab work, and how would you handle this situation?

• Click on **Return to Nurses' Station**.
• Click on **406** to go to Patricia Newman's room.
• Click on **Patient Care** and then **Nurse-Client Interactions**.
• Click on the video titled **0740: Evaluation—Response to Care**. (*Note:* Check the virtual clock to see whether enough time has elapsed. You can use the fast-forward feature to advance the time by 2-minute intervals if the video is not yet available. Then click again on **Patient Care** and **Nurse-Client Interactions** to refresh the screen.)

9. Although Patricia Newman is happy that her chest does not hurt like it did, what does she verbalize as a concern?

10. How does the nurse respond to this expressed concern? Is it an adequate response?

11. When evaluating the care of Patricia Newman, for what potential complications of IV potassium therapy would you monitor? (*Hint:* Consult the Drug Guide provided by clicking on the **Drug** icon in the lower left corner of your screen.)

LESSON 7

Electrolyte Imbalances, Part 2

👓 **Reading Assignment:** Fluid and Electrolyte Balance (Chapter 14)
Interventions for Clients with Electrolyte Imbalances
(Chapter 16)

Patient: Pablo Rodriguez, Room 405

Goal: Utilize the nursing process to competently care for patients with electrolyte imbalances.

Objectives:

1. Describe the pathophysiologic basis of electrolyte imbalances noted on a specific patient.
2. Identify specific etiologic factor(s) related to hypercalcemia, hyponatremia, and hypophosphatemia in the assigned patient.
3. Assess the assigned patient for clinical manifestations related to sodium, calcium, and phosphorus imbalances.
4. Describe nursing interventions appropriate when caring for a patient with hypercalcemia, hyponatremia, and hypophosphatemia.
5. Evaluate the effectiveness of medication prescribed to treat electrolyte imbalances.

In this lesson you will assess, plan, and implement care for a patient with several electrolyte imbalances. Pablo Rodriguez is a 71-year-old male who is admitted with nausea and vomiting for several days. He has a 1-year history of lung carcinoma. You will begin this lesson by reviewing the general functions of specific electrolytes within the body as presented in your textbook. Answer the following questions to cement your understanding of the normal physiologic concepts related to phosphorus, sodium, chloride, and calcium balance.

✏️ **Clinical Preparation: Writing Activity**

 20 minutes

1. Before caring for a client with multiple electrolyte imbalances, it is imperative that you review and reinforce general concepts related to specific electrolytes. Using the textbook, complete the table on the next page with information related to calcium, phosphorus, sodium, and chloride. Refer to this table as you proceed through the CD-ROM exercises to relate textbook knowledge to actual patient care.

89

Electrolyte	Normal Level	Functions	Major Location (i.e., ICF or ECF)	Pathophysiologic Influences
Calcium				
Phosphorus				
Sodium				
Chloride				

CD-ROM Activity

45 minutes

Exercise 1

- Sign in to work at Pacific View Regional Hospital for Period of Care 1. (*Note:* If you are already in the virtual hospital from a previous exercise, click on **Leave the Floor** and then **Restart the Program** to get to the sign-in window.)
- From the Patient List, select Pablo Rodriguez (Room 405).
- Click on **Go to Nurses' Station**.
- Click on **Chart** and then on **405**.
- Click on **Laboratory Reports**.

1. Complete the table below by recording Pablo Rodriguez's serum chemistry results. Identify any abnormal values by marking as H (for high) or L (for low).

Lab Test	Lab Result Tuesday 2000	Lab Result Wednesday 0730
Sodium		
Potassium		
Chloride		
Calcium		
Phosphorus		
Magnesium		

- Click on **Emergency Department** and review this record.

2. What would be the most likely cause for the hyponatremia and hypochloremia noted on admission in this client?

3. What did the physician order to treat this electrolyte imbalance?

4. Find Pablo Rodriguez's sodium and chloride levels for Wednesday at 0730. Was the physician's ordered treatment effective? Are there any changes in physician orders you might anticipate or suggest?

5. Hyponatremia can be associated with both hypovolemia (actual sodium loss) and hypervolumia (dilutional). Initially, in the Emergency Department, what do you think Pablo Rodriguez's volume status was? Explain.

 • Click on **Return to Nurses' Station**.
   • Click on **EPR**.
   • Click on **Login**.
   • Choose **405** from the Patient drop-down menu and select **I&O** as the category.

6. Below, record the I&O shift totals for Pablo Rodriguez.

Shift Totals	Tuesday 0705	Tuesday 1505	Tuesday 2305	Wednesday 0705
Intake				
Output				

7. Based on the above I&O totals obtained after Pablo Rodriguez received IV replacement therapy, what factor(s) do you think may be contributing to the persistent hyponatremia? Explain your answer.

8. What other laboratory tests might be useful to more accurately determine the client's hydration status? (*Hint:* See page 218 in your textbook.)

→ • Click on **Exit EPR**.
  • Click on **405** to go to Pablo Rodriguez's room.
  • Click on **Patient Care** and then **Physical Assessment**.

9. Complete a physical assessment on Pablo Rodriguez, specifically looking for clinical manifestations of hyponatremia. (*Hint:* Refer to textbook page 234.) Document your findings in the table below; underline or highlight those that correlate with hyponatremia.

Areas Assessed	Findings on Physical Examination
Cardiovascular	
Respiratory	
Neuromuscular	
Gastrointestinal	

• Click on **Chart** and then **405**.
• Click on the **Nursing Admission** tab.

10. What other factors could be causing or contributing to the manifestations that you underlined or highlighted in the table in question 9?

11. Based on your answer to questions 9 and 10, what conclusion can you make regarding these clinical manifestations and Pablo Rodriguez's sodium levels?

 12. What other clinical manifestations of hyponatremia might you expect to find in other clients with this electrolyte imbalance? (*Hint:* See textbook pages 234-235.)

13. If Pablo Rodriguez's sodium level were 120 (severe hyponatremia), how would the treatment vary?

CD-ROM Activity

60 minutes

Exercise 2

- Sign in to work at Pacific View Regional Hospital for Period of Care 3. (If you are still in the virtual hospital from Exercise 1, click on **Leave the Floor** and then **Restart the Program** to get to the sign in window.)
- From the Patient List, select Pablo Rodriguez (Room 405).
- Click on **Go to Nurses' Station**.
- Click on **Chart** and then on **405**.
- Click on **Laboratory Reports**.

1. What was Pablo Rodriguez's calcium level on admission to the ED on Tuesday evening?

2. Is this level normal, high, or low?

3. What was his phosphorus level during the same time frame?

4. How does this relate to his calcium level? Explain the pathophysiologic rationale supporting your answer.

5. What other laboratory test(s) would give the nurse a more accurate picture of Pablo Rodriguez's calcium balance? Explain your answer.

6. What is the relationship between Pablo Rodriguez's hyponatremia and hypercalcemia?

 • Click on the **History and Physical** tab of the chart.

7. What would be the most likely cause for Pablo Rodriguez's hypercalcemia? (*Hint:* See Table 16-6 in your textbook.)

 • Click on **Physician's Orders**.

8. What medication did the Emergency Department physician order to treat the hypercalcemia?

9. Describe the mechanism of action of the medication you identified in question 8.

 • Click on **Return to Nurses' Station**.
• Click on the **Drug Guide** on the counter.

10. What nursing assessments are appropriate related to the administration of pamidronate?

 • Click on **Return to Nurses' Station**.
• Click on **Chart** and then on **405**.
• Click on **Laboratory Reports**.

11. What was Pablo Rodriguez's calcium and phosphorus levels this AM (Wednesday at 0730)?

12. Was the prescribed medication effective? Is the client out of danger?

→ • Click on **Return to Nurses' Station**.
  • Click on **Kardex** and then on **405**.

13. What intravenous fluids is Pablo Rodriguez receiving?

14. What is the purpose of IV hydration in relation to serum calcium levels?

15. Is this the normal solution you would expect to administer to a client with hypercalcemia? If not, what solution would you expect and why?

→ • Click on **Return to Nurses' Station**.
  • Click on **MAR** and then on **405**.

16. What medication is scheduled to be administered at 1500?

17. What electrolyte imbalance will this medication correct? Explain your answer. (*Hint:* For help, consult the Drug Guide.)

18. What nursing assessments must be completed before this drug is administered?

19. Do you have any concerns regarding administering this drug at this specific time? (*Hint:* Check the client's GI history on admission.)

- Click on **Return to Nurses' Station**.
- Go to Pablo Rodriguez's room by clicking on **405**.
- Click on **Patient Care** and then **Physical Assessment**.

20. Complete a physical assessment of Pablo Rodriguez (including vital signs) and document your findings below and on the following page.

Areas Assessed	Findings on Physical Examination
Cardiovascular	
Respiratory	

Areas Assessed	**Findings on Physical Examination**

Neuromuscular

Gastrointestinal

21. Is Pablo Rodriguez demonstrating any clinical manifestations of hypercalcemia? If yes, describe the pathophysiologic basis for the symptoms. If not, explain why not.

 22. If Pablo Rodriguez's calcium level was 12.5, what other clinical manifestations might the nurse expect to find? (*Hint:* See page 241 in your textbook.)

23. When evaluating the renal output of Pablo Rodriguez, what potential complication of hypercalcemia would you be alert for?

24. Based on your vascular assessment of Pablo Rodriguez, what complication of hypercalcemia must the nurse vigilantly assess for? Explain.

25. After successful treatment of Pablo Rodriguez, the nurse must be alert for overcorrecting of the electrolyte imbalance. What clinical manifestations should the nurse monitor this client for related to hypocalcemia and hyperphosphatemia?

Acid-Base Imbalance

/∽ **Reading Assignment:** Acid-Base Balance (Chapter 18)
Interventions for Clients with Acid-Base Imbalances
(Chapter 19)

Patients: Jacquline Catanazaro, Room 402
Patricia Newman, Room 406

Goal: Utilize the nursing process to competently care for patients with acid-base imbalances.

Objectives:

1. Describe the pathophysiologic basis of acid-base imbalance noted in assigned patients.
2. Identify specific etiologic factor(s) related to respiratory acidosis in the assigned patients.
3. Assess the assigned patients for clinical manifestations related to respiratory acidosis.
4. Describe nursing interventions appropriate when caring for specific patients with respiratory acidosis.
5. Evaluate the effectiveness of medication prescribed to treat acid-base imbalances.

In this lesson you will assess, plan, and implement care for a patient with an acid-base imbalance. Jacquline Catanazaro is a 45-year-old female admitted with exacerbation of asthma and schizophrenia. Patricia Newman is a 61-year-old female admitted with pneumonia and a 12-year history of emphysema. You will begin this lesson by reviewing the general concepts of acid-base balance as presented in your textbook.

Clinical Preparation: Writing Activity

20 minutes

1. Define the following terms:

   a. Acid

b. Base

c. pH

2. Identify and describe three methods of acid-basis homeostasis by completing the following table.

Line of Defense	Type of Defense	Mechanisms of Action
First line of defense		
Second line of defense		
Third line of defense		

CD-ROM Activity

45 minutes

Exercise 1

- Sign in to work at Pacific View Regional Hospital for Period of Care 1. (*Note:* If you are already in the virtual hospital from a previous exercise, click on **Leave the Floor** and then **Restart the Program** to get to the sign-in window.)
- From the Patient List, select Jacquline Catanazaro (Room 402).
- Click on **Go to Nurses' Station**.
- Click on **Chart** and then on **402**.
- Click on **History and Physical**.

1. Is there anything in Jacquline Catanazaro's history that would put her at risk for an acid-base balance?

- Click on **Return to Nurses' Station**.
- Click on **402**.
- Click on **Patient Care** and then **Nurse-Client Interactions**.
- Select and view the video titled **0730: Intervention—Airway**. (*Note:* Check the virtual clock to see whether enough time has elapsed. You can use the fast-forward feature to advance the time by 2-minute intervals if the video is not yet available. Then click again on **Patient Care** and **Nurse-Client Interactions** to refresh the screen.)

2. Based on Jacquline Catanazaro's history, what would the nurse expect to be causing her respiratory distress?

3. Why is the nurse waiting until after the ABGs are drawn to give the client a nebulizer treatment?

- Click on **Chart** and then on **402**.
- Click on **Laboratory Reports**.

4. What are the results of Jacquline Catanazaro's two most recent ABGs? Document the results in the table below.

Results	Monday 1030	Wednesday 0730
pH		
PaO_2		
$PaCO_2$		
O_2 sat		
Bicarb		

5. How would you interpret the above results? Is the acid-base imbalance compensated or uncompensated (fully or partially)? Explain your answer.

6. Based on the acute aspect of Jacquline Catanazaro's respiratory difficulties, what lines of defense would you expect to be working to compensate for her respiratory acidosis?

7. If the client's electrolyte results were available, what might you expect her potassium levels to be? Provide a rationale for your answer. (*Hint:* See textbook pages 286-287.)

8. Based on Jacquline Catanazaro's medical diagnosis, what is the underlying pathophysiologic problem leading to the respiratory acidosis? (*Hint:* See page 284 of the textbook.)

→ • Click on **Return to Room 402**.
• Click on **Patient Care** and then **Physical Assessment**.

9. Do a complete physical assessment on the client and record your findings below.

Areas Assessed	Findings on Physical Examination
Neurologic	
Musculoskeletal	
Cardiovascular	
Respiratory	
Integumentary	

10. Are there any clinical manifestations of respiratory acidosis? If so, please describe. If not, how do you explain?

➤ • Click on **Take Vital Signs**.

11. What is the client's respiratory rate? How does this correlate with her respiratory acidosis?

12. If Jacquline Catanazaro's pH were 7.2, how might her physical assessment differ? Document the expected clinical manifestations of respiratory acidosis below.

Assessment Area	Expected Findings
Neurologic	
Musculoskeletal	
Cardiovascular	
Respiratory	
Integumentary	

→ • Click on **Chart**.
  • Click on **402** for Jacquline Catanazaro's chart.
  • Click on **Physician's Orders**.

13. Look at the most recent physician's orders. What medication is ordered to treat the respiratory acidosis? What is the medication's underlying mechanism of action to correct the acidosis?

→ • Click on **Return to Room 402**.
  • Click on **Leave the Floor**.
  • Click on **Restart the Program**.
  • Sign in for Period of Care 2.
  • From the Patient List, select Jacquline Catanazaro.
  • Click on **Go to Nurses' Station**.
  • Click on **Chart** and then on **402**.
  • Click on **Laboratory Reports**.

14. Look at the ABGs drawn at 1000. How would you interpret the ABGs? Was the treatment effective?

CD-ROM Activity

45 minutes

Exercise 2

- Sign in to work at Pacific View Regional Hospital for Period of Care 1. (*Note:* If you are already in the virtual hospital from a previous exercise, click on **Leave the Floor** and then **Restart the Program** to get to the sign-in window.)
- From the Patient List, select Patricia Newman (Room 406).
- Click on **Go to Nurses' Station**.
- Click on **Chart** and then on **406**.
- Click on the **History and Physical** tab.

1. Is there anything in Patricia Newman's history that would put her at risk for an acid-base imbalance?

 • Click on **Laboratory Reports**.

2. What are the results of Patricia Newman's two most recent ABGs? Document your findings in the table below.

Results	Tuesday 2300	Wednesday 0500
pH		
PaO_2		
$PaCO_2$		
O_2 sat		
Bicarb		

3. How would you interpret the results you recorded in the previous table? Is the acid-base imbalance compensated or uncompensated (fully or partially)? Explain your answer.

4. Based on the chronic aspect of Patricia Newman's respiratory difficulties, what lines of defense would you expect to be working to compensate for the respiratory acidosis?

5. Based on the ABG results, has Patricia Newman's condition improved or worsened since admission the evening before?

 • Click on **Nurse's Notes**.

6. Read the notes for Wednesday 0730. Describe the actions taken by the nurse. Are they appropriate or not? Explain you answer.

7. What additional actions do you think would be appropriate at this time?

→ • Click on **Laboratory Reports**.

8. What is the client's serum potassium level?

 9. How would you explain the client's hypokalemia in concert with respiratory acidosis? (*Hint:* Check the concurrent medications and page 287 in the textbook.)

10. Based on Patricia Newman's medical diagnosis, what is the underlying pathophysiologic problem leading to the respiratory acidosis? (*Hint:* See page 284 of the textbook.) How does that differ from Jacquline Catanazaro's problem in Exercise 1 of this lesson?

→ • Click on **Return to Nurses' Station** and then **406**.
  • Click on **Patient Care** and then **Physical Assessment**.

11. Do a complete physical assessment, including vital signs, on Patricia Newman. Document your findings below.

Areas Assessed	Findings on Physical Examination
Neurologic	
Musculoskeletal	
Cardiovascular	
Respiratory	
Integumentary	

12. Does Patricia Newman demonstrate any clinical manifestations of respiratory acidosis? If so, please describe. If not, explain why not.

13. What nursing interventions could you, as a graduate nurse, plan and implement to improve Patricia Newman's acid-base balance and prevent complications?

10 _____

Osteoarthritis and Total Knee Replacement

_____

◎⃟ **Reading Assignment:** Interventions for Clients with Connective Tissue Disease and Other Types of Arthritis (Chapter 24)

Patient: Clarence Hughes, Room 404

Goal: Utilize the nursing process to competently care for patients with connective tissue disease.

Objectives:

1. Describe clinical manifestations and treatment of a patient with debilitating osteoarthritis.
2. Document a focused assessment on a postoperative patient who has undergone a total knee arthroplasty.
3. Plan appropriate interventions to prevent complications related to a total knee replacement in an assigned patient.
4. Identify and provide rationales for collaborative care measures used to treat a patient after a total knee arthroplasty.

In this lesson you will learn the essentials of caring for a patient undergoing a total knee arthroplasty for treatment of debilitating osteoarthritis. You will document assessments, plan, implement, and evaluate care given. Clarence Hughes is a 73-year-old male admitted for an elective knee replacement. You will begin this lesson by reviewing the general concepts as presented in your textbook.

✎ **Clinical Preparation: Writing Activity**

⏱ 15 minutes

1. Briefly describe the pathophysiology of osteoarthritis (OA).

2. List causative factors related to the occurrence of primary OA.

3. What are the clinical manifestations of OA?

4. What laboratory and/or radiographic testing is used in the diagnosis of OA?

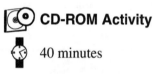

CD-ROM Activity

40 minutes

Exercise 1

- Sign in to work at Pacific View Regional Hospital for Period of Care 1. (*Note:* If you are already in the virtual hospital from a previous exercise, click on **Leave the Floor** and then **Restart the Program** to get to the sign-in window.)
- From the Patient List, select Clarence Hughes (Room 404).
- Click on **Go to Nurses' Station**.
- Click on **Chart** and then on **404**.
- Click on **History and Physical**.

1. Why was Clarence Hughes admitted to the hospital?

2. Describe the symptoms that brought him to this point.

3. According to the H&P, what medications and/or treatments were used to treat Clarence Hughes before he elected to have surgery?

4. Explain the rationale for performing a total knee replacement on this client.

➔ • Click on **Surgical Reports**.

5. How does the report of operation describe the surgical procedure performed on Clarence Hughes?

 6. Based on your reading from the textbook, what can you add to the above description of a total knee arthroplasty?

7. What medication was added to the cement used for this procedure? Explain the rationale for the use of this medication.

8. What was Clarence Hughes' estimated blood loss (EBL)?

 • Click on **Physician's Orders**.
• Scroll down to read the orders for Sunday 1600.

9. What frequent assessments are ordered? Describe specifically how these assessments are completed and what the nurse is looking for.

10. What drain is ordered for Clarence Hughes?

11. What is the expected amount of drainage?

 • Click on **Return to Nurses' Station**.
• Click on **EPR**, then on **Login**.
• Select **404** from the drop-down menu next to Patient.
• Choose **Intake and Output** as the category.

12. Find Drain 1 and review the documentation of hemovac drainage. How much total drainage is recorded?

→ • Click on **Exit EPR**.
 • Now click on **Chart**.
 • Click on **404** for Clarence Hughes' chart.
 • Select the **Physician's Orders** tab.
 • Scroll down to read the orders for Sunday 1600.

13. What is ordered to be applied to the operative knee?

14. What is the purpose of this device? (*Hint:* Your answer to question 13 is a brand name for a hot/ice machine.)

→ • Scroll up to the orders for Monday 0715.

15. What is ordered to prevent knee contractures? Explain the basic use of this device.

16. How should Clarence Hughes' operative leg be positioned during the night? Explain the rationale for this position.

→ • Click on **Laboratory Reports**.

17. What was Clarence Hughes' H&H on Tuesday at 0600?

18. Why do you think his H&H was decreased? (*Hint:* Look at the admitting H&H, EBL, drainage output, and intravenous intake.)

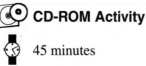 • Click on **Physician's Orders**.

19. What was ordered to correct the above laboratory result?

 CD-ROM Activity

45 minutes

Exercise 2

- Sign in to work at Pacific View Regional Hospital for Period of Care 1. (*Note:* If you are already in the virtual hospital from a previous exercise, click on **Leave the Floor** and then **Restart the Program** to get to the sign-in window.)
- From the Patient List, select Clarence Hughes (Room 404).
- Click on **Get Report**.

1. What are your concerns for Clarence Hughes after receiving report?

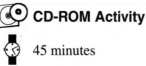 • Click on **Go to Nurses' Station**.
- Click on **404** to go to Clarence Hughes' room.
- Click on **Patient Care** and then **Physical Assessment**.

2. Based on Clarence Hughes' diagnosis and surgery, complete a focused assessment and document your findings below.

Area Assessed	Findings

→ • Click on **Clinical Alerts**.

3. Based on these findings, what would be your priority interventions?

→ • Click on **Medication Room**.

• Click on **MAR** to determine prn medications that have been ordered for Clarence Hughes to address his constipation and pain. (*Note:* You may click on **Review MAR** at any time to verify correct medication order. Remember to look at the patient name on the MAR to make sure you have the correct patient's record—you must click on the correct room number within the MAR. Click on **Return to Medication Room** after reviewing the correct MAR.)

• Click on **Unit Dosage** (or on the Unit Dosage cabinet); from the close-up view, click on drawer **404**.

• Select the medications you would like to administer. After each selection, click **Put Medication on Tray**. When you are finished selecting medications, click **Close Drawer**.

• Click on **View Medication Room**.

• Click on **Automated System** (or on the Automated System unit itself). Click **Login**.

• On the next screen, specify the correct patient and drawer location.

• Select the medication you would like to administer and click on **Put Medication on Tray**. Repeat this process if you wish to administer other medications from the Automated System.

• When you are finished, click **Close Drawer**. At the bottom right corner of the next screen, click on **View Medication Room**.

• From the Medication Room, click on **Preparation** (or on the preparation tray).

• From the list of medications on your tray, choose the correct medication to administer.

• Click **Next**, specify the correct patient to administer this medication to, and click **Finish**.

• Repeat the previous two steps until all medications that you want to administer are prepared.

• You can click on **Review Your Medications** and then on **Return to Medication Room** when ready. Once you are back in the Medication Room, you may go directly to Clarence Hughes' room by clicking on **404** at bottom of screen.

• Administer the medication, utilizing the five rights of medication administration. After you have collected the appropriate assessment data and are ready for administration, click **Patient Care** and then **Medication Administration**. Verify that the correct patient and medication(s) appear in the left-hand window. Then click the down arrow next to Select. From the drop-down menu, select **Administer** and complete the Administration Wizard by providing any information requested. When the Wizard stops asking for information, click **Administer to Patient**. Specify **Yes** when asked whether this administration should be recorded in the MAR. Finally, click **Finish**. You will evaluate your performance in this area at the end of this exercise (see question 14).

4. What is missing on Clarence Hughes' order for oxycodone with acetaminophen? What measures need to be taken?

5. Based on the knowledge that most antacids frequently decrease absorption of other medications when concurrently administered, what options might the nurse employ to ensure adequate absorption of pain medication? (*Hint:* Look in the Drug Guide.)

> • Click on **Patient Care** and then **Nurse-Client Interactions**.
> • Select and view the video titled **0735: Empathy**. (*Note:* Check the virtual clock to see whether enough time has elapsed. You can use the fast-forward feature to advance the time by 2-minute intervals if the video is not yet available. Then click again on **Patient Care** and **Nurse-Client Interactions** to refresh the screen.)

6. The nurse attempts to appear empathetic by offering to listen to the client's concerns. Are her actions congruent with her verbal communication? Why or why not?

7. As a student nurse, what would you do differently?

8. While planning nursing care for Clarence Hughes, identify potential complications related to his postoperative status and measures that can be employed to prevent them. Document your plan of care below.

Complications   **Preventative Measures**

 • Click on **Chart** and then on **404**.
   • Click on **Consultations**.

9. What is physical therapy (PT) doing for Clarence Hughes?

 • Click on **Physician's Orders**.

10. What is the client's activity order for Wednesday morning?

→ • Click on **Nurse's Notes**.

11. What is Clarence Hughes' goal for CPM therapy today?

12. Do you think the ambulation and CPM goals are sufficient for this client to be discharged tomorrow? Why or why not? (*Hint:* Review his home situation in the Nursing Admission form in his chart.)

→ • Click on **Patient Education**.

13. What teaching should be completed for Clarence Hughes before his discharge?

Now let's see how you did during your earlier medication administration!

→ • Click on **Leave the Floor** at the bottom of your screen. From the Floor Menu, select **Look at Your Preceptor's Evaluation**. Then click on **Medication Scorecard**.

14. Disregard the report for the routine scheduled medications but note below whether or not you correctly administered the appropriate prn medications. If not, why do you think you were incorrect? According to Table C in this scorecard, what resources should be used and what important assessments should be completed before administering these medications? Did you utilize these resources and perform these assessments correctly?

Cancer

Reading Assignment: Altered Cell Growth and Cancer Development (Chapter 27)
General Interventions for Clients with Cancer (Chapter 28)
Interventions for Clients with Noninfectious Problems of the
Lower Respiratory Tract (Chapter 33, pages 613-625)

Patient: Pablo Rodriguez, Room 405

Goal: Utilize the nursing process to competently care for patients with cancer.

Objectives:

1. Describe clinical manifestations and treatment for a patient with cancer.
2. Recognize special needs of patients undergoing treatment for cancer.
3. Appropriately treat a patient's symptoms related to disease process and/or side effects of treatment.
4. Discuss medications prescribed for an assigned patient, including expected therapeutic effects as well as adverse/side effects to monitor for.
5. Plan appropriate general interventions to prevent and/or treat complications related to chemotherapy.

In this lesson you will learn the essentials of caring for a patient diagnosed with cancer. You will collect data, assess, plan, implement, and evaluate care given. Pablo Rodriguez is a 71-year-old male admitted with advanced non-small-cell lung carcinoma. You will begin this lesson by reviewing the general concepts of cancer as presented in your textbook.

Clinical Preparation: Writing Activity

20 minutes

1. Define the following terms:

a. Carcinogenesis

    b. Oncogene

    c. Nadir

2. What are the three types of therapies used to treat cancer? Describe their respective mechanisms of action.

3. What are the four most common side effects of chemotherapy?

4. What are some common side effects associated with radiation therapy?

5. Identify the common sites of distant metastasis for lung cancer.

6. List the warning signals associated with lung cancer. (*Hint:* See Table 33-9 in textbook.)

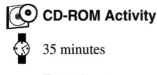 **CD-ROM Activity**

35 minutes

Exercise 1

- Sign in to work at Pacific View Regional Hospital for Period of Care 1. (*Note:* If you are already in the virtual hospital from a previous exercise, click on **Leave the Floor** and then **Restart the Program** to get to the sign-in window.)
- From the Patient List, select Pablo Rodriguez (Room 405).
- Click on **Go to Nurses' Station**.
- Click on **Chart** and then on **405** for Pablo Rodriguez's chart.
- Click on **History and Physical**.

1. What is Pablo Rodriguez's main diagnosis?

2. How long ago was he diagnosed?

3. What risk factor for lung cancer is documented on the H&P?

4. What are other risk factors for lung cancer? (*Hint:* See pages 613-614 of your textbook.)

5. What clinical manifestations documented in the physician's review of systems are related to this disease process?

6. What treatment has Pablo Rodriguez received so far?

7. How long ago did he receive his last chemotherapy?

8. What are the mechanism of action and the major side effects of docetaxel? (*Hint:* For help, return to the Nurses' Station and click on the **Drug Guide** on the counter.)

9. What is the nadir of docetaxel? Would Pablo Rodriguez still be having side effects from this drug? Explain.

10. What specific assessments related to potential bone marrow suppression should the nurse monitor? What interventions are appropriate to prevent complications of bone marrow suppression?

→ • Click on **Physician's Notes** in the chart.

11. Look at the notes for Tuesday 1800. What type of cancer is noted? Is this the same as or different from the non-small-cell cancer noted in the H&P? Explain.

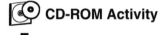 **CD-ROM Activity**

🕐 30 minutes

Exercise 2

• Sign in to work at Pacific View Regional Hospital for Period of Care 1. (*Note:* If you are already in the virtual hospital from a previous exercise, click on **Leave the Floor** and then **Restart the Program** to get to the sign-in window.)
• From the Patient List, select Pablo Rodriguez (Room 405).
• Click on **Get Report** and read the change-of-shift report.

1. What unresolved problem for Pablo Rodriguez is noted in the report?

→ • Click on **Go to Nurses' Station**.
• Click on **Chart** and then on **405** for Pablo Rodriguez's chart.
• Click on **Nurse's Notes**.

2. Look at the note for Wednesday at 0415. How did the nurse respond to Pablo Rodriguez's complaints? Were the nurse's actions appropriate?

3. How might you have responded differently?

→ • Click on **Return to Nurses' Station**.
  • Go to Pablo Rodriguez's room by clicking on **405**.
  • Click on **Patient Care** and then **Nurse-Client Interactions**.
  • Select and view the video titled **0735: Patient Perceptions**. (*Note:* Check the virtual clock to see whether enough time has elapsed. You can use the fast-forward feature to advance the time by 2-minute intervals if the video is not yet available. Then click again on **Patient Care** and **Nurse-Client Interactions** to refresh the screen.)

  4. What are Pablo Rodriguez's two major concerns at this point?

  5. What other assessment should you perform before treating client's complaint of nausea?

→ • Click on **MAR**; then select tab **405** to access Pablo Rodriguez's record.

  6. What medications are ordered to manage the client's pain and nausea?

  7. What might the nurse question regarding these medication orders?

→ • Click on **Return to Room 405**.
  • Click on **Chart**.
  • Click on **405** for the correct chart.
  • Click on **Nursing Admission**.

  8. What is the client's weight? What is this in kgs?

→ • Click on **Return to Room 405**.
  • Click on the **Drug** icon in the lower left corner of the screen.

9. Calculate the maximum 24-hour dose for clients receiving this drug for nausea related to chemotherapy.

10. Calculate the maximum 24-hour dose of this drug for management of postoperative nausea and vomiting.

11. Calculate the maximum amount of metoclopramide Pablo Rodriguez could receive per 24 hours as ordered. Is this within the dosage guidelines? Is there any reason to be concerned about this dosage schedule over long periods of time?

12. What are the possible ramifications of giving high doses of this drug?

13. What are the ramifications of *not* giving metoclopramide for this client's complaint of nausea?

14. If the nurse administers the prn Reglan at 0730, what should be done with the regularly scheduled 0800 dose?

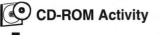 **CD-ROM Activity**

40 minutes

Exercise 3

- Sign in to work at Pacific View Regional Hospital for Period of Care 2. (*Note:* If you are already in the virtual hospital from a previous exercise, click on **Leave the Floor** and then **Restart the Program** to get to the sign-in window.)
- From the Patient List, select Pablo Rodriguez (Room 405).
- Click on **Go to Nurses' Station**.
- Click on **Chart** and then on **405** for Pablo Rodriguez's chart.
- Click on **Laboratory Reports**.

1. In the table below, record Pablo Rodriguez's alkaline phosphatase and calcium levels.

Lab Result	Tuesday 2000	Wednesday 0730
Alkaline phosphatase		
Calcium		

2. How do these abnormal results relate to the client's diagnosis of cancer?

 • Click on **Emergency Department** and review this record.

3. What is Pablo Rodriguez's chief complaint on admission to the ED? How is this related to his cancer? (*Hint:* Read the ED physician's progress notes for Tuesday at 1800.)

 • Click on **Return to Nurses' Station**.
- Click on **MAR** and then on tab **405** to access Pablo Rodriguez's records.

4. What medications still need to be given to Pablo Rodriguez for the day shift (up to 1500)?

➥ • Click on **Return to Nurses' Station**.
  • Click on the **Drug** icon in the lower left corner of the screen.
  • Use the Drug Guide to answer the next three questions.

  5. How does ondansetron differ from metoclopramide in regard to antiemetic mechanism of action?

  6. Over what period of time would you infuse the IV ondansetron?

  7. What is the expected benefit that Pablo Rodriguez will receive from dexamethasone? Over how many minutes should it be administered?

➥ • Click on **Return to Nurses' Station**.
  • Click on **Chart** and then on **405** for Pablo Rodriguez's chart.
  • Click on **Patient Education**.

  8. Has any teaching yet been completed? In your opinion, what priority teaching should have been completed upon admission?

  • Click on **Return to Nurses' Station**.
  • Go to Pablo Rodriguez's room by clicking on **405**.
  • Click on **Patient Care** and then **Nurse-Client Interactions**.
  • Select and view the video titled **1150: Assessment—Pain**. (*Note:* Check the virtual clock to see whether enough time has elapsed. You can use the fast-forward feature to advance the time by 2-minute intervals if the video is not yet available. Then click again on **Patient Care** and **Nurse-Client Interactions** to refresh the screen.)

9. Why is Pablo Rodriguez not eating?

10. Is this a normal side effect of chemotherapy?

11. How would you treat this?

➤ • Click on **Kardex** and select tab **405**. Read the outcomes.

12. What additional outcome(s) might you include for this client?

13. What is Pablo Rodriguez's code status? How do you feel about this in relation to his diagnosis and condition? What is the nurse's professional responsibility related to the client's code status?

LESSON **12** ————————————————————————

Asthma

————————————————————————

👓 **Reading Assignment:** Interventions for Clients with Noninfectious Problems of the
Lower Respiratory Tract (Chapter 33)

Patient: Jacquline Catanazaro, Room 402

Goal: Utilize the nursing process to competently care for patients with asthma.

Objectives:

1. Identify clinical manifestations of an acute asthmatic exacerbation.
2. Evaluate diagnostic tests as they relate to a patient's oxygenation status.
3. Identify medications used to treat asthma, along with their mechanism of action and therapeutic effects.
4. Prioritize nursing care for a patient with an acute exacerbation of asthma.
5. Formulate an appropriate patient education plan regarding home asthma management for a
   patient with identified barriers to learning.

In this lesson you will learn the essentials of caring for a patient diagnosed with asthma. You
will explore the patient's history, evaluate presenting symptoms and treatment on admission, and
follow the patient's progress throughout the hospital stay. Jacquline Catanazaro is a 45-year-old
female admitted with increasing respiratory distress. You will begin this lesson by reviewing the
general concepts of asthma as presented in your textbook.

✒ **Clinical Preparation: Writing Activity**

⏱ 30 minutes

1. Briefly describe the pathophysiology of asthma.

149

2. What category of lung diseases does asthma belong to?

3. In the table below, compare and contrast the four steps of asthma management.

Stages of Asthma Management	Clinical Manifestations	Treatment Recommendations
Mild intermittent		
Mild persistent		
Moderate persistent		
Severe persistent		

4. Define the following pulmonary function tests measurements:

a. Forced vital capacity (FVC)

b. Forced expiratory volume in the first second (FEV_1)

c. Peak expiratory flow rate (PEFR)

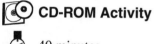 **CD-ROM Activity**

40 minutes

Exercise 1

- Sign in to work at Pacific View Regional Hospital for Period of Care 1. (*Note:* If you are already in the virtual hospital from a previous exercise, click on **Leave the Floor** and then **Restart the Program** to get to the sign-in window.)
- From the Patient List, select Jacquline Catanazaro (Room 402).
- Click on **Go to Nurses' Station**.
- Click on **Chart** and then on **402** for Jacquline Catanazaro's chart.
- Click on **History and Physical**.

1. What medical problems does Jacquline Catanazaro have?

2. What pathologic triggers can lead to an exacerbation of asthma?

3. Does Jacquline Catanazaro's history identify any of these triggers?

4. What other factor(s) might be contributing to her asthma exacerbations?

5. Based on Jacquline Catanazaro's history and home medication regimen, what step of asthma management do you think she is normally at (disregarding this admission for an exacerbation)? Explain.

→ • Click on **Emergency Department** and review this record.

6. What were Jacquline Catanazaro's presenting symptoms?

7. What diagnostic testing was ordered? Record and interpret the abnormal results below. (*Hint:* Click on **Laboratory Reports** and **Diagnostic Reports** to obtain the results.)

8. Read the ED physician's progress notes for 1400. What are the results of Jacquline Catanazaro's PEFR? How would you interpret these in light of her present condition?

➡ • Click on **Physician's Orders**.

9. What medical treatment is ordered in the ED? (*Hint:* See the orders for Monday at 1005.)

10. How would you evaluate the client's response to medical treatment?

11. What medications were ordered on Monday at 1600? What is the mechanism of action for each of these medications? (*Hint:* Click on **Return to Nurses' Station**; then click on the **Drug Guide** on the counter or on the **Drug** icon in the lower left corner of your screen.)

12. In what order would the nurse administer these medications? Provide a rationale.

13. What new medications are ordered on Tuesday at 0800? Give a rationale for these orders. Why is the prednisone ordered to be decreased by 5 mg every day?

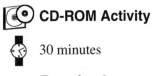 **CD-ROM Activity**

30 minutes

Exercise 2

- Sign in to work at Pacific View Regional Hospital for Period of Care 1. (*Note:* If you are already in the virtual hospital from a previous exercise, click on **Leave the Floor** and then **Restart the Program** to get to the sign-in window.)
- From the Patient List, select Jacquline Catanazaro (Room 402).
- Click on **Go to Nurses' Station**.
- Click on **402** to go to the client's room.
- Click on **Initial Observations**.

1. Describe your initial observations when you enter Jacquline Catanazaro's room.

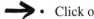 • Click on **Take Vital Signs**.

2. Record Jacquline Catanazaro's vital signs below.

3. Are there any clinical alerts for Jacquline Catanazaro? If so, describe below.

4. How would you prioritize your care for this client at this point?

→ • Click on **Patient Care** and then **Physical Assessment**.

5. Perform and document a focused assessment on three priority areas based on Jacquline Catanazaro's present status. Identify these areas and record your findings below.

Focused Areas of Assessment	Jacquline Catanazaro's Assessment Findings

→ • Click on **Chart** and then on **402** for Jacquline Catanazaro's chart.
 • Click on **Physician's Orders**.

6. What new orders did the physician write on Monday at 0730?

- Click on **Return to Room 402**.
- Click on **Patient Care** and then **Nurse-Client Interactions**.
- Select and view the video titled **0730: Intervention—Airway**. (*Note:* Check the virtual clock to see whether enough time has elapsed. You can use the fast-forward feature to advance the time by 2-minute intervals if the video is not yet available. Then click again on **Patient Care** and **Nurse-Client Interactions** to refresh the screen.)

7. How does this nurse prioritize her actions? What reasons can you give for her actions?

- Click on **Clinical Alerts**.

8. Look at the 0800 clinical alert. Give your interpretation of this alert.

- Click on **Chart** and then on **402**.
- Click on **Physician's Notes**.

9. Read the notes for Wednesday at 0800. How does the physician evaluate the client's condition at this point?

- Click on **Physician's Orders**. Find the orders for 0800 on Wednesday.

10. Record each order below and provide a rationale for each.

New Orders	Rationale/Expected Therapeutic Response

CD-ROM Activity

45 minutes

Exercise 3

- Sign in to work at Pacific View Regional Hospital for Period of Care 2. (*Note:* If you are already in the virtual hospital from a previous exercise, click on **Leave the Floor** and then **Restart the Program** to get to the sign-in window.)
- From the Patient List, select Jacquline Catanazaro (Room 402).
- Click on **Get Report**.

1. Briefly summarize the activity for Jacquline Catanazaro over the last 4 hours.

- Click on **Go to Nurses' Station**.
- Click on **402** to go to Jacquline Catanazaro's room.
- Click on **Initial Observations**.

2. What is your initial observation of the client for this time period?

3. Are there any clinical alerts?

- Click on **Take Vital Signs**.

4. How do the results of these vital signs compare with those you obtained during Period of Care 1? (*Hint:* See Exercise 2, question 2 for those findings.)

• Click on **Patient Care** and then **Physical Assessment**.

5. Perform a focused assessment on Jacquline Catanazaro. Record you findings below. Then compare the results with your assessment during Period of Care 1 and interpret your results. (*Hint:* For your earlier assessment findings, see Exercise 2, question 5.)

Focused Areas of Assessment	Current Findings	Comparison with Earlier Findings—Interpretation of Results

 • Click on **Patient Care** and then **Nurse-Client Interactions**.
   • Select and view the video titled **1115: Assessment—Readiness to Learn**. (*Note:* Check the virtual clock to see whether enough time has elapsed. You can use the fast-forward feature to advance the time by 2-minute intervals if the video is not yet available. Then click again on **Patient Care** and **Nurse-Client Interactions** to refresh the screen.)

6. Describe the nurse's actions in the video. Are they appropriate? Explain.

7. What barriers to learning might be present for Jacquline Catanazaro?

 • Click on **Chart** and then on **402** for Jacquline Catanazaro's chart.
 • Click on **Patient Education**.

8. What are the educational goals for Jacquline Catanazaro?

9. What other asthma management needs would you teach the client? (*Hint:* See Chart 33-4 in your textbook on page 589.)

10. Describe the differences in outcomes met for Jacquline Catanazaro and her sister.

11. The client is scheduled for discharge tomorrow. Do you have any concerns? What would be your most appropriate action?

→ • Click on **Return to Room 402**.
 • Click on **Leave the Floor**.
 • Choose to **Restart the Program**.
 • Sign in to work at Pacific View Regional Hospital for Period of Care 3.
 • From the Patient List, select Jacquline Catanazaro (Room 402).
 • Click on **Go to Nurses' Station**.
 • Click on **402**.
 • Select **Patient Care** and then **Nurse-Client Interactions**.
 • Select and view the video titled **1500: Intervention—Patient Teaching**. (*Note:* Check the virtual clock to see whether enough time has elapsed. You can use the fast-forward feature to advance the time by 2-minute intervals if the video is not yet available. Then click again on **Patient Care** and **Nurse-Client Interactions** to refresh the screen.)

12. What equipment is the nurse teaching the client about?

13. Describe the proper use of the peak flow meter for clients.

 14. Describe the preferred technique of use for a metered dose inhaler (MDI). (*Hint:* See Chart 33-6 on page 593 of your textbook.)

Emphysema and Pneumonia

/ORO **Reading Assignment:** Interventions for Clients with Noninfectious Problems of the Lower Respiratory Tract (Chapter 33)

Interventions for Clients with Infectious Problems of the Lower Respiratory Tract (Chapter 34)

Patient: Patricia Newman, Room 406

Goal: Utilize the nursing process to competently care for patients with altered oxygenation states.

Objectives:

1. Relate physical assessment findings with pathophysiologic changes of the lower respiratory tract.
2. Prioritize nursing care for a patient with altered oxygenation.
3. Evaluate laboratory results relative to the diagnosis of pneumonia and emphysema.
4. Describe pharmacologic interventions related to altered oxygenation states.
5. Identify appropriate nursing interventions for a patient admitted with pneumonia and emphysema.
6. Identify appropriate discharge teaching needs for a patient with altered oxygenation.

In this lesson you will learn the essentials of caring for a patient diagnosed with pneumonia and emphysema. You will explore the patient's history, evaluate presenting symptoms and treatment upon admission, and assess the patient's progress throughout the hospital stay. Patricia Newman is a 61-year-old female admitted with pneumonia and a history of emphysema. You will begin this lesson by reviewing the general concepts of altered oxygenation states as presented in your textbook.

Clinical Preparation: Writing Activity

20 minutes

1. What category(ies) of lung diseases does emphysema belong to?

2. Briefly describe the pathophysiology of emphysema.

3. Briefly describe the pathophysiology of pneumonia.

4. What are the risk factors for community-acquired pneumonia?

CD-ROM Activity

45 minutes

Exercise 1

- Sign in to work at Pacific View Regional Hospital for Period of Care 1. (*Note:* If you are already in the virtual hospital from a previous exercise, click on **Leave the Floor** and then **Restart the Program** to get to the sign-in window.)
- From the Patient List, select Patricia Newman (Room 406).
- Click on **Get Report**.

1. What questions would you ask the outgoing nurses to obtain needed information that was not identified in report?

2. Below, relate the clinical manifestations identified in the report to the client's diagnosis of pneumonia by identifying the pathophysiologic basis of each manifestation.

Clinical Manifestations	Pathophysiologic Basis
Labored respirations	
Use of accessory muscles	
Productive cough with yellow sputum	
Coarse breath sounds	
Lung infiltrates	
Disturbed sleep patterns	
Tachycardia	
Fever	

• Click on **Go to Nurses' Station**.
  • Click on **Chart** and then on **406** for Patricia Newman's chart.
  • Click on **History and Physical**.

3. What risk factors for community-acquired pneumonia does Patricia Newman have?

 • Click on **Nursing Admission**.

4. What other risk factor for community-acquired pneumonia is documented on this form?

 • Click on **Return to Nurses' Station**.
  • Click on **406** to enter Patricia Newman's room.
  • Click on **Initial Observation**.

5. What would be your priority nursing assessment/intervention(s) based on your initial observations of Patricia Newman?

 • Click on **Patient Care** and then **Physical Assessment**. Perform a focused assessment based on her admitting diagnosis.

6. Record your findings below. How has Patricia Newman's condition changed since report?

Focused Assessment Area	Assessment Findings	Change in Assessment

→ • Click on **Patient Care** and then **Nurse-Client Interactions**.

• Select and view the video titled **0730: Prioritizing Interventions**. (*Note:* Check the virtual clock to see whether enough time has elapsed. You can use the fast-forward feature to advance the time by 2-minute intervals if the video is not yet available. Then click again on **Patient Care** and **Nurse-Client Interactions** to refresh the screen.)

7. Evaluate the nurse's actions based on the client's current status. How does this nurse's action differ from your plan of care as answered in question 5 of this exercise?

8. What nursing interventions might be done to alleviate the client's anxiety?

→ • Click on **Chart** and then on **406** for Patricia Newman's chart.

• Click on **Laboratory Reports**.

9. Identify any abnormal laboratory results and describe how they correlate with Patricia Newman's diagnosis of pneumonia.

→ • Click on **Return to Room 406**.

• Click on **MAR**.

10. What is the desired therapeutic effect of ipratoprium bromide? How could the nurse assess whether the desired effect was achieved?

11. What is the desired therapeutic effect of cefotetan? How could the nurse assess whether the desired effect was achieved?

12. What is the rationale for administration of IV fluids related to pneumonia?

- Click on **Medication Room**.
- Click on **MAR** to determine medications that Patricia Newman is ordered to receive at 0800 and any appropriate prn medications you may want to administer. (*Note:* You may click on **Review MAR** at any time to verify correct medication order. Remember to look at the patient name on the MAR to make sure you have the correct patient's record—you must click on the correct room number within the MAR. Click on **Return to Medication Room** after reviewing the correct MAR.)
- Click on **Unit Dosage**. When the close-up view appears, click on drawer **406**.
- Select the medication(s) you plan to administer. After each medication you select, click **Put Medication on Tray**. When you are finished, click on **Close Drawer**.
- Click **View Medication Room**.
- Click on **IV Storage**. From the close-up view, click on the drawer labeled **Large Volume**.
- Select the medication(s) you plan to administer, put medication(s) on tray, and close bin.
- Click **View Medication Room**.
- Click on **Preparation**. Select the correct medication to administer; click **Prepare** and **Next.**
- Choose the correct patient to administer this medication to and click **Finish**.
- Repeat the above two steps until all medications that you want to administer are prepared.
- You can click **Review Your Medications** and then **Return to Medication Room** when ready. From the Medication Room, you may go directly to Patricia Newman's room by clicking on **406** at bottom of screen.
- Administer the medication, utilizing the five rights of medication administration. After you have collected the appropriate assessment data and are ready for administration, click **Patient Care** and then **Medication Administration**. Verify that the correct patient and medication(s) appear in the left-hand window. Then click the down arrow next to Select. From the drop-down menu, select **Administer** and complete the Administration Wizard by providing any information requested. When the Wizard stops asking for information, click **Administer to Patient**. Specify **Yes** when asked whether this administration should be recorded in the MAR. Finally, click **Finish**.

Now let's see how you did!

- Click on **Leave the Floor** at the bottom of your screen. From the Floor Menu, select **Look at Your Preceptor's Evaluation**. Then click on **Medication Scorecard**.

13. Note below whether or not you correctly administered the appropriate medications. If not, why do you think you were incorrect? According to Table C in this scorecard, what are the appropriate resources that should be used and important assessments that should be completed before administering these medications? Did you use these resources and perform these assessments correctly?

CD-ROM Activity

40 minutes

Exercise 2

- Sign in to work at Pacific View Regional Hospital for Period of Care 2. (*Note:* If you are already in the virtual hospital from a previous exercise, click on **Leave the Floor** and then **Restart the Program** to get to the sign-in window.)
- From the Patient List, select Patricia Newman (Room 406).
- Click on **Go to Nurses' Station**.
- Click on **Chart** and then on **406** for Patricia Newman's chart.
- Click on **History and Physical**.

1. For how long has Patricia Newman been diagnosed with emphysema?

2. What clinical manifestations documented on the H&P can be attributed to emphysema?

3. What additional clinical manifestations might you expect to see in other clients with emphysema?

→ - Click on **Diagnostic Reports**.

4. What findings on the CXR are consistent with the diagnosis of emphysema?

5. What is the relationship between the client's admitting diagnosis (pneumonia) and her underlying chronic condition (emphysema)?

• Click on **Physician's Orders**.

   6. What is the order for oxygen?

   7. What is the rationale for this oxygen order as opposed to the usual goal of greater than 90% to 93% oxygen saturation?

 • Click on **Patient Education**.

   8. What is educational goal 3 for Patricia Newman?

   9. Explain the rationale for using this technique and describe how you would teach the client to achieve goal 3. (*Hint:* See Chart 33-10 on page 603 in your textbook.)

  10. What is educational goal 4 for Patricia Newman?

11. What do you think Patricia Newman's special dietary needs are? Explain your answer.

12. What is educational goal 6 for Patricia Newman?

13. What is the rationale for using this technique? How would you teach Patricia Newman to cough effectively?

 14. Since Patricia Newman's emphysema puts her at high risk for pulmonary infections, what would you teach her to do to help prevent further episodes of pneumonia? (*Hint:* See Chart 34-4 on page 634 of your textbook.)

→ • Click on **Return to Nurses' Station**.
  • Click on **406** to go to Patricia Newman's room.
  • Choose **Patient Care** and then **Nurse-Client Interactions**.
  • Select and view the video titled **1100: Care Coordination**. (*Note:* Check the virtual clock to see whether enough time has elapsed. You can use the fast-forward feature to advance the time by 2-minute intervals if the video is not yet available. Then click again on **Patient Care** and **Nurse-Client Interactions** to refresh the screen.)

15. What disciplines are involved in planning and providing care for Patricia Newman? List these in the left column below. In the right column, explain the role of each person in helping meet the client's health care needs.

Involved Disciplines	Role in Patricia Newman's Health Care

Pulmonary Embolism

Reading Assignment: Interventions for Critically Ill Clients with Respiratory Problems (Chapter 35)

Patient: Clarence Hughes, Room 404

Goal: Utilize the nursing process to competently care for patients with a critically altered oxygenation state.

Objectives:

1. Identify clinical manifestations of pulmonary embolism.
2. Prioritize nursing care for a patient with acute onset of respiratory distress and chest pain.
3. Describe diagnostic testing relative to the diagnosis of pulmonary embolism.
4. Describe pharmacologic therapy for patient with a pulmonary embolism.
5. Accurately calculate correct dosage of heparin for patient using a sliding scale.
6. Identify disease management issues regarding the care of a patient with a pulmonary embolism.

In this lesson you will learn the essentials of caring for a patient diagnosed with an acute pulmonary embolism. You will explore the patient's history, evaluate presenting symptoms and treatment, provide appropriate nursing interventions, and assess the patient's progress throughout the clinical day. Clarence Hughes is a 73-year-old-male admitted for an elective left knee arthroplasty.

CD-ROM Activity

30 minutes

Exercise 1

- Sign in to work at Pacific View Regional Hospital for Period of Care 2. (*Note:* If you are already in the virtual hospital from a previous exercise, click on **Leave the Floor** and then **Restart the Program** to get to the sign-in window.)
- From the Patient List, select Clarence Hughes (Room 404).
- Click on **Get Report**.

1. Before entering Clarence Hughes' room, summarize what you would expect to find based on the report you received.

 • Click on **Go to Nurses' Station**.
• Click on **404** to go to Clarence Hughes' room.

2. What is your initial observation as you enter the client's room?

3. What should your priority actions be at this point?

 • Click on **Patient Care** and then **Nurse-Client Interactions**.
• Select and view the video titled **1115: Interventions—Airway**. (*Note:* Check the virtual clock to see whether enough time has elapsed. You can use the fast-forward feature to advance the time by 2-minute intervals if the video is not yet available. Then click again on **Patient Care** and **Nurse-Client Interactions** to refresh the screen.)

4. Describe the nursing actions in the video. Was it appropriate for the nurse to leave the client to go get oxygen? Why or why not? If not, what else could she have done?

5. What classic signs and symptoms of pulmonary embolus is Clarence Hughes displaying?

6. Suspecting a pulmonary embolus, what other clinical manifestations would you assess for in Clarence Hughes? (*Hint:* See Chart 35-2 on page 651 of textbook.)

• Click on **Chart** and then on **404** for Clarence Hughes' chart.
• Click on **History and Physical**.

7. Based on the client's history and the current reason for hospitalization, what risk factors for DVT and resultant pulmonary embolus does Clarence Hughes have?

• Click on **Physician's Orders**.

8. Look at the orders dated Wednesday at 1120. Document these orders below and provide a rationale for each order.

Physician Order	Rationale

➔ • Click on **Return to Room 404**.

• Click on **Patient Care** and then **Nurse-Client Interactions**.

• Select and view the video titled **1135: Change in Patient Condition**. (*Note:* Check the virtual clock to see whether enough time has elapsed. You can use the fast-forward feature to advance the time by 2-minute intervals if the video is not yet available. Then click again on **Patient Care** and **Nurse-Client Interactions** to refresh the screen.)

9. As the nurse is explaining care to the family, she states that a transporter will be coming to take Clarence Hughes for a ventilation-perfusion scan. Would you send this client down to radiology with just the transporter? Why or why not?

CD-ROM Activity

30 minutes

Exercise 2

• Sign in to work at Pacific View Regional Hospital for Period of Care 3. (*Note:* If you are already in the virtual hospital from a previous exercise, click on **Leave the Floor** and then **Restart the Program** to get to the sign-in window.)

• From the Patient List, select Clarence Hughes (Room 404).

• Click on **Go to Nurses' Station**.

• Click on **Chart** and then on **404** for Clarence Hughes' chart.

• Select and review the **Laboratory Reports** and **Diagnostic Reports** sections of the chart.

1. Below, document the results of the ordered diagnostic testing.

Diagnostic Test	**Result**

2. Based on the above results, what would you conclude to be the cause of Clarence Hughes' acute respiratory distress?

➤ • Click on **Physician's Orders**.

    3. What orders were written to treat Clarence Hughes' pulmonary embolus?

    4. What laboratory test will be used to titrate the heparin infusion? What are the normal values for this test?

    5. What is the desired therapeutic level for this laboratory test?

➤ • Click on **Return to Nurses' Station**.
    • Click on **MAR** and then on **404** for Clarence Hughes' record.

    6. How many mL of heparin would you administer for the bolus dose?

    7. If you were the nurse starting the heparin infusion, at what rate would you set the IV pump to infuse this medication?

➤ • Click on **Return to Nurses' Station**.
    • Click on **Chart** and then on **404** for Clarence Hughes' record.
    • Click on **Laboratory Reports**.

8. What were the results of the aPTT and INR at 1300 today? Why were these tests ordered prior to starting the heparin?

➡ • Click on **Return to Nurses' Station**.
   • Click on **404** to enter Clarence Hughes' room.
   • Click on **Patient Care** and then **Nurse-Client Interactions**.
   • Select and view the video titled **1510: Disease Management**. (*Note:* Check the virtual clock to see whether enough time has elapsed. You can use the fast-forward feature to advance the time by 2-minute intervals if the video is not yet available. Then click again on **Patient Care** and **Nurse-Client Interactions** to refresh the screen.)

9. When the son asks the nurse whether the pulmonary embolism will delay his father's discharge, the nurse states that the heparin takes 2 days to stabilize. Does this mean that the client will be discharged on heparin? If not, what medication will be used to minimize clot formation? Explain why the client is not started on this medication rather than heparin.

10. What lab test(s) will be used to monitor the therapeutic effect of Coumadin? What is the therapeutic range for these tests?

11. For what possible complications would you monitor Clarence Hughes related to the pulmonary embolism?

CD-ROM Activity

30 minutes

Exercise 3

- Sign in to work at Pacific View Regional Hospital for Period of Care 4. (*Note:* If you are already in the virtual hospital from a previous exercise, click on **Leave the Floor** and then **Restart the Program** to get to the sign-in window.)
- Click on **Chart** and then on **404** for Clarence Hughes' chart. (*Remember:* You are not able to visit patients or administer medications during Period of Care 4. You are able to review patients' records only.)
- Click on **Laboratory Reports**.

  1. What is the aPTT result for 1900?

 • Click on **Return to Nurses' Station**.
- Click on **MAR** and then on **404** for Clarence Hughes' record.

  2. What would you do now with the heparin infusion? Calculate the correct infusion rate and document below. (*Hint:* Refer to your answer for question 6 in Exercise 2.)

 • Click on **Return to Nurses' Station**.
- Click on **Kardex** and then on **404** for Clarence Hughes' record.

  3. Are there any additional outcomes that should be added based on the client's current setback? Give a rationale.

4. If the heparin was not effective in treating Clarence Hughes and his conditioned worsened, what other pharmacological treatment might be helpful? Explain.

5. Describe bleeding precautions that must be followed while this client is receiving heparin therapy.

6. If Clarence Hughes' condition deteriorates, what surgical treatment might be needed? Explain.

7. If this client develops another pulmonary embolism, what further treatment might the physician consider to prevent the recurrence of PEs? Explain.

LESSON **15**

Atrial Fibrillation

👓 **Reading Assignment:** Interventions for Clients with Dysrhythmias (Chapter 37)

Patient: Piya Jordan, Room 403

Goal: Utilize the nursing process to competently care for patients with atrial fibrillation.

Objectives:

1. Describe telemetry rhythm strip characteristics of atrial fibrillation.
2. Identify potential etiologic causes of atrial fibrillation for an assigned patient.
3. Assess a patient for clinical manifestations of atrial fibrillation.
4. Develop plan of care to monitor a patient for potential complications of atrial fibrillation.
5. Perform appropriate assessments prior to administering pharmacologic therapy for atrial fibrillation.
6. Accurately administer IV digoxin.
7. Discuss the use of anticoagulation therapy for a patient with atrial fibrillation.
8. Develop appropriate educational outcomes for a patient with a history of atrial fibrillation.

In this lesson you will learn the essentials of caring for a patient with a cardiac dysrhythmia. You will explore the patient's history, evaluate presenting symptoms and treatment, provide appropriate nursing interventions, and plan an appropriate patient educational outcomes related to the dysrhythmia. Piya Jordan is a 68-year-old female admitted with nausea, vomiting, and abdominal pain.

✒ **Clinical Preparation: Writing Activity**

🕐 20 minutes

1. Describe the normal conduction system of the heart.

179

2. Describe the concept of atrial-ventricular synchrony. Why is this important?

3. Identify the cardiac event represented by each of the following waves and measured intervals:

a. P wave

b. QRS wave

c. T wave

d. PR interval

e. QT interval

f. U wave

4. Describe the six steps of ECG analysis.

 CD-ROM Activity

35 minutes

Exercise 1

- Sign in to work at Pacific View Regional Hospital for Period of Care 1. (*Note:* If you are already in the virtual hospital from a previous exercise, click on **Leave the Floor** and then **Restart the Program** to get to the sign-in window.)
- From the Patient List, select Piya Jordan (Room 403).
- Click on **Go to Nurses' Station**; then click on **403** to enter the client's room.

1. What information regarding Piya Jordan's cardiovascular status is obtained on initial observation?

2. What is telemetry monitoring?

3. What is atrial fibrillation?

4. Describe the rhythm strip you would expect to see on Piya Jordan's monitor.

5. How does this differ from normal sinus rhythm?

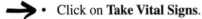

 • Click on **Take Vital Signs**.

6. Record Piya Jordan's heart rate below and state whether the rhythm is controlled or uncontrolled atrial fibrillation. Explain your answer.

7. For what clinical manifestations related to atrial fibrillation should you monitor?

→ • Click on **Patient Care** and then **Physical Assessment** to perform a general assessment of Piya Jordan.

8. Are any of the symptoms you identified in question 7 present in this client? If not, how can you explain that?

9. If Piya Jordan's heart rate increases, how might the atrial fibrillation affect her blood pressure? Describe the underlying physiology. (*Hint:* Think about normal atrial-ventricular synchrony.)

→ • Click on **Chart** and then on **403**.

• Click on the **Diagnostic Reports** tab.

10. Did Piya Jordan have a 12-lead ECG done? If yes, what was the rhythm? If not, do you think it should have been done? Why or why not?

11. For what potential complications should you monitor Piya Jordan?

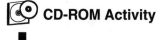 **CD-ROM Activity**

45 minutes

Exercise 2

• Sign in to work at Pacific View Regional Hospital for Period of Care 1. (*Note:* If you are already in the virtual hospital from a previous exercise, click on **Leave the Floor** and then **Restart the Program** to get to the sign-in window.)

• From the Patient List, select Piya Jordan (Room 403).

• Click on **Go to Nurses' Station**.

• Click on **MAR** and then on tab **403**.

1. What medication is prescribed to treat Piya Jordan's atrial fibrillation? Describe the pharmacodynamics of this medication as related to atrial fibrillation. (*Hint:* You may need to consult the Drug Guide.)

2. Why did the physician order a digoxin level when the client first presented to the ED? (*Hint:* Look at client's presenting symptoms as well as the Drug Guide.)

• Click on **Return to Nurses' Station**.
   • Click on **Chart** and then on **403**.
   • Click on **Laboratory Reports**.

3. What was Piya Jordan's digoxin level in the ED? Is this therapeutic or toxic?

4. For what other symptoms would you monitor Piya Jordan in relation to digoxin toxicity?

5. What was her potassium level on admission to the Emergency Department?

6. How does this relate to possible digoxin toxicity?

• Click on **History and Physical**.

7. What other medication was Piya Jordan prescribed related to atrial fibrillation prior to this admission? Explain the rationale for this medication. (*Hint:* Think of potential serious complications of atrial fibrillation.)

• Click on **Physician's Orders**.

8. What two items did the physician prescribe preoperatively to reverse Piya Jordan's anticoagulation? How would you know whether this was effective? Explain.

9. What was ordered postoperatively to prevent clot formation?

→ • Click on **Nursing Admission**.

10. What knowledge (or lack of knowledge) does Piya Jordan verbalize regarding her history of atrial fibrillation? (*Hint:* Look at the Health Promotion section.)

→ • Click on **Patient Education**.

11. What might you add to these outcomes based on your answer to question 10?

12. How would treatment for Piya Jordan differ if her atrial fibrillation was a new acute onset?

13. What surgical treatment options may be used for clients with recurrent or sustained atrial fibrillation?

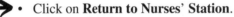

- Click on **Return to Nurses' Station**.
- Click on **Medication Room**.
- Click on **MAR** to determine medications that Piya Jordan is ordered to receive at 0800. (*Note:* You may click on **Review MAR** at any time to verify correct medication order. Remember to look at the patient name on the MAR to make sure you have the correct patient's record—you must click on the correct room number within the MAR. Click on **Return to Medication Room** after reviewing the correct MAR.)
- Based on your care for Piya Jordan, access the various storage areas of the Medication Room to obtain the necessary medications you need to administer.
- For each area you access, first select the medication you plan to administer, then click **Put Medication on Tray**. When finished with a storage area, click on **Close Drawer**.
- Click **View Medication Room**.
- Click on **Preparation** and choose the correct medication to administer. Click **Prepare**.
- Click **Next** and choose the correct patient to administer this medication to. Click **Finish**.
- Repeat the above two steps until all medications that you want to administer are prepared.
- You can click **Review Your Medications** and then **Return to Medication Room** when you are ready. Once you are back in the Medication Room, you may go directly to Piya Jordan's room by clicking on **403** at the bottom of the screen.
- Administer the medication, utilizing the five rights of medication administration. After you have collected the appropriate assessment data and are ready for administration, click **Patient Care** and then **Medication Administration**. Verify that the correct patient and medication(s) appear in the left-hand window. Then click the down arrow next to Select. From the drop-down menu, select **Administer** and complete the Administration Wizard by providing any information requested. When the Wizard stops asking for information, click **Administer to Patient**. Specify **Yes** when asked whether this administration should be recorded in the MAR. Finally, click **Finish**.

14. Over how many minutes would you administer the IV digoxin?

15. What should you have assessed prior administering digoxin to Piya Jordan today?

Now let's see how you did!

→ • Click on **Leave the Floor** at the bottom of your screen. From the Floor Menu, select **Look at Your Preceptor's Evaluation**. Then click on **Medication Scorecard**.

16. Note below whether or not you correctly administered the appropriate medication(s). If not, why do you think you were incorrect? According to Table C in this scorecard, what resources should be used and what important assessments should be completed before administering the medication(s)? Did you utilize these resources and perform these assessments correctly?

Hypertension

/O⊂⊃ **Reading Assignment:** Interventions for Clients with Vascular Problems (Chapter 39)

Patients: Patricia Newman, Room 406
Harry George, Room 401

Goal: Utilize the nursing process to competently care for patients with hypertension.

Objectives:

1. Describe the four classifications of blood pressure.
2. Identify the presence of risk factors for hypertension in assigned patients.
3. Discuss pharmacologic therapies available to treat hypertension.
4. Perform appropriate assessments prior to administering pharmacologic therapy for hypertension.
5. Develop an extensive educational plan for patients with hypertension.

In this lesson you will learn the essentials of caring for a patient with hypertension. You will explore the patient's history, evaluate presenting symptoms and treatment, identify blood pressure classification, provide appropriate nursing interventions, and plan an appropriate patient educational plan related to the hypertension. Patricia Newman is a 61-year-old female admitted with pneumonia and a history of emphysema. Harry George is a 54-year-old male admitted with infection and swelling of the left foot.

Clinical Preparation: Writing Activity

20 minutes

1. Identify and describe the four classifications of blood pressure.

   a.

   b.

   c.

   d.

2. Identify and describe the three physiologic controls of blood pressure.

   a.

   b.

   c.

3. Define the following terms:

   a. Malignant hypertension

   b. Secondary hypertension

   c. Orthostatic hypotension

4. List the risk factors for essential hypertension.

   a.

   b.

   c.

   d.

   e.

   f.

   g.

   h.

   i.

   j.

   k.

   l.

CD-ROM Activity

45 minutes

Exercise 1

- Sign in to work at Pacific View Regional Hospital for Period of Care 1. (*Note:* If you are already in the virtual hospital from a previous exercise, click on **Leave the Floor** and then **Restart the Program** to get to the sign-in window.)
- From the Patient List, select Patricia Newman (Room 406).
- Click on **Go to Nurses' Station**.
- Click on **Chart** and then on **406** to access the correct chart.
- Click on **History and Physical**.

1. How long has Patricia Newman been diagnosed with hypertension?

→ • Click on **Nursing Admission**.

2. What risk factors for hypertension does she have?

➔ • Click on **Physician's Orders**.

3. In the left column of the table below, list all medications ordered to treat Patricia Newman's hypertension. For each medication, identify the drug classification and its mechanism of action. (*Note:* You will complete the table in questions 4 and 5.)

Medication	Drug Classification	Mechanism of Action	Nursing Assessments	Side Effects

4. What nursing assessments are important before administering each of these medications? Record your answers in the fourth column of the table above.

5. For what side effects will the nurse need to monitor the client? Record you answer in the last column of the table above. (*Hint:* You may also use your textbook as a resource.)

6. What are Patricia Newman's documented blood pressure measurements since admission?

7. Is her prescribed antihypertensive medication currently effective? Explain.

8. In what classification of blood pressure would you place Patricia Newman based on her most current readings? Explain your decision.

9. What might be contributing to her currently elevated blood pressure?

10. What indicates that Patricia Newman is in need of further teaching regarding hypertension?

11. What additional educational goals would be appropriate for this client?

12. Develop a comprehensive teaching plan for Patricia Newman regarding nonpharmacologic measures and interventions to treat hypertension.

13. Was Patricia Newman following any of the above interventions to reduce her blood pressure at home? Explain.

14. Identify any of the interventions you addressed in question 12 that were ordered for Patricia Newman during this hospital stay.

15. As the nurse caring for Patricia Newman, what do you think would be your professional responsibility related to your findings for questions 13 and 14?

CD-ROM Activity

40 minutes

Exercise 2

- Sign in to work at Pacific View Regional Hospital for Period of Care 1. (*Note:* If you are already in the virtual hospital from a previous exercise, click on **Leave the Floor** and then **Restart the Program** to get to the sign-in window.)
- From the Patient List, select Harry George (Room 401).
- Click on **Go to Nurses' Station**.
- Click on **EPR** and then on **Login**.
- Choose **401** from the drop-down menu next to Patient. Select **Vital Signs** as the category.

1. Document Harry George's blood pressures for the times specified below.

	Tues 0305	**Tues 0705**	**Tues 1105**	**Tues 1505**
BP reading				

	Tues 1905	**Tues 2305**	**Wed 0305**	**Wed 0705**
BP reading				

2. Does Harry George have a history of hypertension?

3. Does he have any risk factors for hypertension? If yes, please identify.

4. Based on the BP recordings in question 1, in what classification would you put Harry George's blood pressure?

5. What potential complications should you assess for related to untreated hypertension?

→ • Click on **Exit EPR**.
  • Click on **Chart** and then **401**.
  • Click on **Physician's Orders**.

6. Several diagnostic tests were ordered by the physician. Although these tests may have been ordered for various purposes, they might specifically help to identify target organ disease. In the middle column below, indicate how each of the listed tests might be helpful. (*Note:* You will complete the table in questions 7 and 8.)

Diagnostic Test	How Test Might Help Identify Target Organ Disease	Results
Chest x-ray		
BUN		
Creatinine		
Urinalysis		

 • Click on **Diagnostic Reports**.

7. Record the result of the chest x-ray in the third column of the table above and indicate whether the results suggest the presence of target organ disease.

→ • Click on **Laboratory Reports.**

8. Find and record the laboratory results for BUN, creatinine, and urinalysis in the table above. Indicate what these results mean related to target organ disease.

9. In the table below, identify the various classifications of hypertensive medications that might be used to treat Harry George's elevated blood pressure. For each classification, briefly describe the mechanism of action.

Drug Classification	Mechanism of Action
a.	
b.	
c.	
d.	
e.	
f.	
g.	
h.	
i.	
j.	

10. What symptoms might Harry George display if his blood pressure dramatically increased above 200 mm Hg?

11. How would you respond if a hypertensive crisis occurred?

LESSON **17** —————————————————————————

Blood Transfusions

✍ **Reading Assignment:** Interventions for Clients with Hematologic Problems (Chapter 43)

Patient: Piya Jordan, Room 403

Goal: Utilize the nursing process to competently care for patients receiving various blood products.

Objectives:

1. Describe the ABO and Rh antigen systems.
2. Identify the correct type blood to administer to a specific patient.
3. Describe appropriate nursing responsibilities related to blood product administration.
4. Evaluate vital sign assessments related to potential blood transfusion reactions.
5. Describe appropriate assessment parameters when monitoring for various types of transfusion reactions.

In this lesson you will learn the essentials of caring for a patient receiving blood and blood product transfusions. You will describe pretransfusion responsibilities, identify administration specifics, and evaluate the patient during and after each transfusion. Piya Jordan is a 68-year-old female admitted with nausea, vomiting, and abdominal pain.

✒ **Clinical Preparation: Writing Activity**

🕐 10 minutes

1. Describe the ABO antigen system.

2. Describe the Rh antigen system.

3. Complete the table below to identify which types of blood are compatible with each other. (*Hint:* Use Table 43-7 in your textbook, reading the recipient blood type at top of column and looking down the column to see what donor type each recipient can receive.)

Client's Blood Type	Blood Types This Client May Receive
A+	
A–	
B+	
B–	
O+	
O–	
AB+	
AB–	

CD-ROM Activity

30 minutes

Exercise 1

- Sign in to work at Pacific View Regional Hospital for Period of Care 1. (*Note:* If you are already in the virtual hospital from a previous exercise, click on **Leave the Floor** and then **Restart the Program** to get to the sign-in window.)
- From the Patient List, select Piya Jordan (Room 403).
- Click on **Go to Nurses' Station,** then on **Chart,** and then on **403**.
- Click on **Laboratory Reports**.

1. Document the results of Piya Jordan's hematology tests below.

	Monday 2200	Tuesday 0630	Wednesday 0630
Hemoglobin			
Hematocrit			

2. Why do you think Piya Jordan's H&H is lower on Wednesday? (*Hint:* Check the Physician's Notes in the chart.)

⮕ • Click on **Physician's Orders**.

3. What was ordered to correct this? Is this appropriate related to Piya Jordan's level of hemoglobin? Explain why or why not.

⮕ • Click on **Return to Nurses' Station**.
  • Click on **403** to enter Piya Jordan's room.
  • Select **Patient Care** and then **Nurse-Client Interactions**.
  • Select and view the video titled **0735: Pain—Adverse Drug Event**. (*Note:* Check the virtual clock to see whether enough time has elapsed. You can use the fast-forward feature to advance the time by 2-minute intervals if the video is not yet available. Then click again on **Patient Care** and **Nurse-Client Interactions** to refresh the screen.)

4. What does the nurse state she will do to prepare Piya Jordan for a blood transfusion?

5. What gauge IV would you insert for the blood transfusion?

6. What other pretransfusion responsibilities would you complete? Have these been completed? (*Hint:* Look in the chart.)

⮕ • Click on **Chart** and then on **403**.
  • Click on **Laboratory Reports**.

7. What day and time was the cross-match completed? According to your textbook, is this laboratory result acceptable for blood being transfused today?

8. Explain how you would prepare the blood set-up prior to administration.

 CD-ROM Activity

30 minutes

Exercise 2

- Sign in to work at Pacific View Regional Hospital for Period of Care 2. (*Note:* If you are already in the virtual hospital from a previous exercise, click on **Leave the Floor** and then **Restart the Program** to get to the sign-in window.)
- From the Patient List, select Piya Jordan (Room 403).
- Click on **Go to Nurses' Station** and then on **403** to enter Piya Jordan's room.
- Click on **Patient Care** and then on **Nurse-Client Interactions**.
- Select and view the video titled **1115: Interventions—Nausea, Blood**. (*Note:* Check the virtual clock to see whether enough time has elapsed. You can use the fast-forward feature to advance the time by 2-minute intervals if the video is not yet available. Then click again on **Patient Care** and **Nurse-Client Interactions** to refresh the screen.)

1. Piya Jordan's daughter verbalizes concern regarding the safety of blood transfusion. How did the nurse respond to this?

2. Describe how you would explain the safety of blood transfusions.

3. During the video, the nurse states that the blood has just arrived. How soon should the nurse begin the transfusion?

→ • Click on **Chart** and then on **403**.
  • Click on **Laboratory Reports**.

4. What is Piya Jordan's blood type?

5. What type of blood may she receive safely?

6. Describe the nurse's responsibilities during the initiation of this transfusion.

7. How fast would you transfuse this unit of blood? Give your rationale.

8. What assessments should be completed on Piya Jordan during the transfusion?

9. What would you document regarding this blood transfusion?

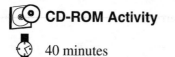 **CD-ROM Activity**

40 minutes

Exercise 3

- Sign in to work at Pacific View Regional Hospital for Period of Care 4. (*Note:* If you are already in the virtual hospital from a previous exercise, click on **Leave the Floor** and then **Restart the Program** to get to the sign-in window.)
- Click on **EPR** and then **Login**. (*Remember:* You are not able to visit patients or administer medications during Period of Care 4. You are able to review patients' records only.)
- Choose **403** from the drop-down menu next to Patient; select **Vital Signs** as the category.

1. Below, record Piya Jordan's vital signs after each of the two units of blood.

	1130	1145	1200	1215	1315	1400	1415	1430	1445	1500	1515	1530
Temp												
Pulse												
BP												
Resp												

2. According to the above vital sign assessments, did Piya Jordan have any adverse reactions to the blood transfusions? Explain.

3. What type of symptoms would you expect to see if Piya Jordan had a hemolytic transfusion reaction?

4. How would these symptoms differ if she had an allergic transfusion reaction?

5. How can you determine that Piya Jordan did not have a febrile reaction if she was febrile at the beginning of the transfusion?

6. What is Piya Jordan's total intake and output over the last 24 hours (i.e., Tuesday at 1500 through Wednesday at 1500)?

→ • Click on **Exit EPR**.
  • Click on **MAR** and then on **403** to access the correct records.

7. Over what period of time was the first unit of RBC infused? Was this appropriate? Explain.

8. What signs and/or symptoms would you expect to see if Piya Jordan was suffering from circulatory overload?

→ • Click on **Return to Nurses' Station**.
 • Click on **Chart** and then on **403** to access Piya Jordan's chart.
 • Click on **Expired MARs**.

9. What other blood product has she received this admission? (*Hint:* Look at Tuesday's MAR.)

10. How does this product differ from RBCs, and why was it given to Piya Jordan? (*Hint:* Look at the History and Physical to determine the reason for giving it.)

11. How does administration of FFP differ from administration of RBCs?

LESSON **18** _____

Lumbosacral Back Pain

_____

👓 **Reading Assignment:** Interventions for Clients with Problems of the Central Nervous System: The Spinal Cord (Chapter 46)

Patient: Jacquline Catanazaro, Room 402

Goal: Utilize the nursing process to competently care for a patient with an intervertebral disk problem.

Objectives:

1. Describe the pathophysiology of low back pain.
2. Identify clinical manifestations related to low back pain and/or herniated intervertebral disk.
3. Plan appropriate interventions to treat low back pain.
4. Evaluate a patient's potential to comply with a health care management plan.
5. Develop an individualized teaching plan for a patient with low back pain.

In this lesson you will learn the essentials of caring for a patient experiencing chronic low back pain. You will explore the patient's history, evaluate presenting symptoms and treatment, plan appropriate nursing interventions to treat the patient's symptoms, and develop an individualized discharge teaching plan. Jacquline Catanazaro is a 45-year-old female admitted with an acute exacerbation of asthma.

✒ **Clinical Preparation: Writing Activity**

🕐 15 minutes

1. Describe the underlying pathophysiology of low back pain.

2. What differentiates acute low back pain from chronic low back pain?

3. Define the following procedures:

  a. Diskectomy

  b. Laminectomy

  c. Spinal fusion (arthodesis)

  d. Percutaneous lumbar diskectomy

  e. Microdiskectomy

  f. Laser-assisted laparoscopic lumbar diskectomy

CD-ROM Activity

45 minutes

Exercise 1

- Sign in to work at Pacific View Regional Hospital for Period of Care 3. (*Note:* If you are already in the virtual hospital from a previous exercise, click on **Leave the Floor** and then **Restart the Program** to get to the sign-in window.)
- From the Patient List, select Jacquline Catanazaro (Room 402).
- Click on **Go to Nurses' Station**.
- Click on **Chart** and then on **402**.
- Click on **History and Physical**.

1. Under "History of Present Illness," what are the client's complaints related to her back?

2. How does the physician describe this problem under "Past Medical History"?

3. How was this diagnosed?

4. How long has Jacquline Catanazaro had this problem?

5. What treatment has she undergone? Explain the mechanism of action and/or rationale for these treatments.

→ • Click on **Nursing Admission**.

6. What risk factor(s) does Jacquline Catanazaro have for low back pain and/or herniated disk disease?

7. What assessments should be completed on this client in relation to the back pain?

→ • Click on **Nurse's Notes**.

8. How have the nurses addressed Jacquline Catanazaro's complaint of low back pain?

9. What interventions could you suggest that would be appropriate for this client's situation?

→ • Click on **History and Physical**.

 10. What is the physician's plan regarding this client's back pain? What type of interventions might be offered by this consult? (*Hint:* See textbook Chapter 7 for interventions.)

11. If Jacquline Catanazaro's pain is not relieved by nonsurgical management, which of the procedures defined in your clinical preparation would you expect to be used for her? Why?

→ • Click on **Patient Education**.

12. What goals related to Jacquline Catanazaro's back pain would you add?

13. Develop a discharge teaching plan for her to help relieve and prevent further back pain.

→ • Click on **History and Physical**.

14. What may interfere with Jacquline Catanazaro's compliance to health care instructions?

→ • Click on **Return to Nurses' Station**.
   • Click on **402** to enter Jacquline Catanazaro's room.
   • Click on **Patient Care** and then **Nurse-Client Interactions**.
   • Select and view the video titled **1540: Discharge Planning**. (*Note:* Check the virtual clock to see whether enough time has elapsed. You can use the fast-forward feature to advance the time by 2-minute intervals if the video is not yet available. Then click again on **Patient Care** and **Nurse-Client Interactions** to refresh the screen.)

15. After viewing the video, what other suggestions do you have for assisting Jacquline Catanazaro with compliance after discharge? (*Hint:* Refer to textbook Chapter 1.)

Glaucoma

 Reading Assignment: Interventions for Clients with Eye and Vision Problems
(Chapter 50)

Patients: Clarence Hughes, Room 404

Goal: Utilize the nursing process to competently care for patients with glaucoma.

Objectives:

1. Describe the pathophysiology of glaucoma.
2. Identify clinical manifestations related to glaucoma.
3. Describe appropriate pharmacologic treatment of glaucoma.
4. Administer eye drops safely and accurately.
5. Evaluate a patient's ability to correctly administered prescribed ophthalmic medication.

In this lesson you will learn the essentials of caring for a patient diagnosed with glaucoma. You will explore the patient's history, evaluate presenting symptoms and treatment, administer prescribed medications, and develop an individualized discharge teaching plan. Clarence Hughes is a 73-year-old male admitted for an elective left knee arthroplasty.

Clinical Preparation: Writing Activity

15 minutes

1. Describe the pathophysiology of glaucoma.

2. Compare and contrast the different types of glaucoma by completing the following table. (*Note:* Disregard any section of the table with an X through it.)

Type of Glaucoma	Etiology	Pathophysiology	Clinical Manifestations
Primary			
Open-angle			
Closed-angle			
Secondary			
Associated			

3. Describe three diagnostic assessments used to diagnose glaucoma.

    a.

    b

    c.

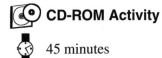 **CD-ROM Activity**

45 minutes

Exercise 1

- Sign in to work at Pacific View Regional Hospital for Period of Care 3. (*Note:* If you are already in the virtual hospital from a previous exercise, click on **Leave the Floor** and then **Restart the Program** to get to the sign-in window.)
- From the Patient List, select Clarence Hughes (Room 404).
- Click on **Go to Nurses' Station**.
- Click on **Chart** and then on **404**.
- Click on **History and Physical**.

1. What problem of the eye does Clarence Hughes have?

2. How would this problem be diagnosed?

3. What signs and symptoms do you think Clarence Hughes had prior to diagnosis?

4. What clinical manifestation should you now assess for related to this diagnosis?

5. The History and Physical does not identify the type of glaucoma Clarence Hughes has. Based on his history and information in the textbook, which type do you think he mostly likely has? Explain why you came to this conclusion.

➤ • Click on **Return to Nurses' Station**.
   • Click on **MAR** and then on **404** to access the correct record.

6. What medications are ordered for Clarence Hughes' glaucoma? Identify these medications, their classifications, and mechanisms of action below. (*Note:* You will complete the last column in question 7.)

Medication	Drug Classification	Mechanism of Action	Side Effects

7. For what side effects should you monitor Clarence Hughes related to these medications? Record your answer in the table above.

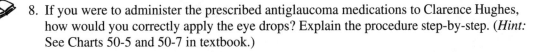

8. If you were to administer the prescribed antiglaucoma medications to Clarence Hughes, how would you correctly apply the eye drops? Explain the procedure step-by-step. (*Hint:* See Charts 50-5 and 50-7 in textbook.)

9. What range of IOP would Clarence Hughes have had prior to beginning treatment for glaucoma? What would you expect his reading to be during treatment?

→ • Click on **Return to Nurses' Station**.
   • Click on **Chart** and then on **404** for Clarence Hughes' chart.
   • Click on **Patient Education**.

10. What educational goals would you add for Clarence Hughes related to his glaucoma?

11. What teaching would you provide to this client regarding his glaucoma?

12. Complete the following table by documenting teaching points you would you review with Clarence Hughes regarding each of his glaucoma medications.

Medication	Teaching Points

13. What teaching methods would you use to teach medication administration to this client?

14. How would you evaluate Clarence Hughes' understanding of correct application?

15. If his ophthalmic medications would fail to maintain IOP within normal limits, what other therapy might Clarence Hughes expect to undergo?

Osteoporosis

✎ **Reading Assignment:** Interventions for Clients with Musculoskeletal Problems
(Chapter 54)

Patients: Patricia Newman, Room 406

Goal: Utilize the nursing process to competently care for patients with osteoporosis.

Objectives:

1. Describe the pathophysiology of osteoporosis.
2. Assess the patient for clinical manifestations of osteoporosis.
3. Describe appropriate pharmacologic therapy for prevention and/or treatment of osteo-porosis.
4. Administer medications safely and accurately.
5. Plan appropriate interventions to promote health and prevent further bone loss in a patient with osteoporosis.
6. Develop an individualized teaching plan for an assigned patient with osteoporosis.

In this lesson you will learn the essentials of caring for a patient diagnosed with osteoporosis. You will explore the patient's history, evaluate presenting symptoms and treatment, administer prescribed medications, and develop an individualized discharge teaching plan. Patricia Newman is a 61-year-old female admitted with pneumonia and a history of emphysema.

✐ **Clinical Preparation: Writing Activity**

🕐 15 minutes

1. Define the following terms:

   a. Bone mineral density (BMD)

b. T-score

c. Osteopenia

d. Osteoclastic

e. Osteoblastic

2. Describe the pathophysiology of osteoporosis.

3. In the table below, compare and contrast the different classifications of osteoporosis.

Classification	Etiology/Description
Generalized	
Primary	
Secondary	
Regional	

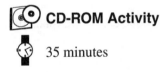 **CD-ROM Activity**

35 minutes

Exercise 1

- Sign in to work at Pacific View Regional Hospital for Period of Care 2. (*Note:* If you are already in the virtual hospital from a previous exercise, click on **Leave the Floor** and then **Restart the Program** to get to the sign-in window.)
- From the Patient List, select Patricia Newman (Room 406).
- Click on **Go to Nurses' Station**.
- Click on **Chart** and then on **406**.
- Click on **History and Physical**.

1. How long has Patricia Newman been diagnosed with osteoporosis?

2. What risk factors does she have for osteoporosis? Are any of these risks modifiable? If so, which ones?

3. What diagnostic test would have been ordered to diagnose Patricia Newman's osteoporosis? Describe the test and the result that would indicate osteoporosis.

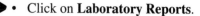 • Click on **Laboratory Reports**.

4. Do any laboratory results for this client correlate with osteoporosis?

5. What other laboratory results should you review in relation to bone density? Explain the relationship between these tests and osteoporosis.

 • Click on **Nursing Admission**.

6. Are there any other risk factors found here?

7. What clinical manifestation of osteoporosis is documented on this form?

8. For what other clinical manifestations would you assess Patricia Newman in relation to osteoporosis?

- Click on **Return to Nurses' Station**.
- Click on **MAR** and then on **406** for the correct records.

9. What medications are ordered for Patricia Newman to help treat and prevent worsening of her osteoporosis? In the table below, identify these medications, their classifications, and mechanisms of action. (*Note:* You will complete the last column in question 10.)

Medication	Drug Classification	Mechanism of Action	Side Effects

10. For what side effects should you monitor the client related to these medications? Record your answer in the table above.

11. If you were to administer the prescribed estradiol to Patricia Newman, how and where would you apply it? Are there any precautions you should take while applying this?

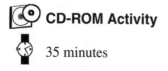

CD-ROM Activity

35 minutes

Exercise 2

- Sign in to work at Pacific View Regional Hospital for Period of Care 3. (*Note:* If you are already in the virtual hospital from a previous exercise, click on **Leave the Floor** and then **Restart the Program** to get to the sign-in window.)
- From the Patient List, select Patricia Newman (Room 406).
- Click on **Go to Nurses' Station**.
- Click on **Chart** and then on **406**.
- Click on **Patient Education**.

1. What educational goals already identified could be applied to this client's osteoporosis?

2. What teaching would you provide Patricia Newman regarding exercise to prevent further bone loss? What other exercises might benefit her?

3. What dietary needs does Patricia Newman have related to the osteoporosis? What foods would you teach her to include in her diet?

4. Complete the following chart to document teaching points you would you review with Patricia Newman regarding her medications to treat osteoporosis.

Medication	Teaching Points

5. Consider this scenario: Patricia Newman asks you what further treatment would be available to her if her bone loss continued despite her present regimen. How would you answer her? (*Hint:* Identify five other drug classifications that might be useful to this client and describe their mechanism of action.)

6. What is Patricia Newman most at risk for related to her osteoporosis?

7. What can you teach her that would help prevent this from occurring at home?

 • Click on **Return to Nurses' Station**.
  • Click on **406** to enter Patricia Newman's room.
  • Click on **Patient Care** and then **Nurse-Client Interactions**.
  • Select and view the video titled **1500: Discharge Planning**. (*Note:* Check the virtual clock to see whether enough time has elapsed. You can use the fast-forward feature to advance the time by 2-minute intervals if the video is not yet available. Then click again on **Patient Care** and **Nurse-Client Interactions** to refresh the screen.)

8. Although this discussion was related to Patricia Newman's pulmonary disease, how would smoking cessation benefit her musculoskeletal problem?

9. What other health care disciplines might be useful to help Patricia Newman with her discharge needs related to osteoporosis?

10. What psychosocial nursing diagnosis might be a potential problem for Patricia Newman related to her slightly stooped posture and going home on oxygen? What nursing interventions would be appropriate to help the client with this difficulty?

Osteomyelitis

Reading Assignment: Interventions for Clients with Musculoskeletal Problems
(Chapter 54)

Patient: Harry George, Room 401

Goal: Utilize the nursing process to competently care for patients with osteomyelitis.

Objectives:

1. Describe the pathophysiology of osteomyelitis.
2. Assess an assigned patient for clinical manifestations of osteomyelitis.
3. Describe the causative agent and category of osteomyelitis in an assigned patient.
4. Safely administer IV antibiotic therapy as prescribed for osteomyelitis.
5. Evaluate diagnostic tests related to osteomyelitis.
6. Develop an individualized discharge plan of care of a patient with osteomyelitis complicated by other disease processes and homelessness.

In this lesson you will learn the essentials of caring for a patient diagnosed with osteomyelitis. You will explore the patient's history, evaluate presenting symptoms and treatment, administer prescribed medications, and develop an individualized discharge teaching plan. Harry George is a 54-year-old male admitted with infection and swelling of his left foot, as well as a history of type 2 diabetes, alcohol abuse, and nicotine addiction.

Clinical Preparation: Writing Activity

10 minutes

1. Describe the pathophysiology of osteomyelitis.

2. Define the following categories of osteomyelitis:

a. Exogenous

b. Endogenous/hematogenous

c. Contiguous

d. Chronic

3. What is the most common causative organism of osteomyelitis?

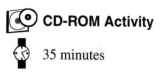 **CD-ROM Activity**

35 minutes

Exercise 1

- Sign in to work at Pacific View Regional Hospital for Period of Care 2. (*Note:* If you are already in the virtual hospital from a previous exercise, click on **Leave the Floor** and then **Restart the Program** to get to the sign-in window.)
- From the Patient List, select Harry George (Room 401).
- Click on **Go to Nurses' Station**.
- Click on **Chart** and then on **401** for Harry George's chart.
- Click on **History and Physical**.

1. The clinical manifestations of osteomyelitis can include both local and systemic symptoms. Common local and systemic signs and symptoms are listed below. Circle signs and symptoms consistent with Harry George's history and physical examination findings on admission.

Local Symptoms	Systemic Symptoms
Severe bone pain	Fever
Swelling	Night sweats
Warmth at infection site	Chills
Restricted movement	Restlessness
	Nausea
	Malaise

2. Based on what you have read, identify the source of Harry George's osteomyelitis and the type (category) of invasion responsible for it. Explain the rationale for your conclusion.

3. What factors in Harry George's history may have contributed to the development of osteomyelitis? (*Hint:* See page 1173 of textbook.)

→ • Click on **Physician's Orders**.

4. The following diagnostic tests are useful in the diagnosis and evaluation of osteomyelitis. Match each test with its corresponding description. Then circle Yes or No to indicate whether each diagnostic test was performed as part of Harry George's admissions work-up.

Diagnostic Test	**Description**
_____ MRI and CT scan (Yes / No)	a. Initial test to determine causative organism
_____ Wound culture (Yes / No)	b. Identifies most cases of osteomyelitis
_____ White blood cell count (Yes / No)	c. Most definitive way to determine causative organism
_____ X-ray of affected extremity (Yes / No)	d. Elevated results of this test indicate infection
_____ Radionuclide bone scan (Yes / No)	e. Radiologic test that is most sensitive in the diagnosis of osteomyelitis
_____ Bone/tissue biopsy (Yes / No)	f. Changes with this test do not appear early in the course of the disease
_____ Erythrocyte sedimentation rate (ESR) (Yes / No)	g. May be normal early in the course of the disease but rises and remains elevated for as long as 3 months after drug therapy is discontinued

→ • Click on **Diagnostic Reports**.

5. Compare these reports with the pathophysiology of osteomyelitis as described in the textbook. What findings documented on these reports are consistent with osteomyelitis? What do these findings mean? Record you answers below.

Finding documented on the x-ray report

Finding documented on the bone scan

Meaning of both

→ • Click on **Return to Nurses' Station**.
   • Click on **MAR** and select tab **401** for Harry George's records.

6. Determine what routine medications (excluding the continuous IV and insulin coverage) you will be giving to Harry George during the day shift (0700-1500). Below, list the medications you need to give, the drug classification, the reason why each drug is given, and the time each is due. (*Hint:* You may refer to the Drug Guide by returning to the Nurses' Station and then clicking on the **Drug** icon in the lower left corner of the screen.)

Medication	Classification	Reason for Giving	Time Due

7. Which medication was Harry George receiving that was discontinued on Tuesday?

→ • Click on **Return to Nurses' Station**.
   • Click on **Chart** and then on **401** for Harry George's chart.
   • Click on **Physician's Orders**.

8. What replaced the medication you identified in question 7?

→ • Click on **Physician's Notes**.

9. Why was this change ordered?

→ • Click on **Laboratory Reports**.

10. You are aware that the antibiotics have been ordered for Harry George because of his leg infection. You decide to check the WBC results because you are curious (also, you are sure your nursing instructor will ask you about it). Document the WBC results for the times specified below. Explain what the results mean, including the direction of the change in the WBC and the significance of this change.

Tests	Mon 1500	Tues 1100	Normal, Elevated, or Decreased?
Total WBC			
Neutrophil Segs			
Neutrophil Bands			
Lymphocytes			
Monocytes			
Eosinophils			
Basophils			

→ • Click on **Return to Nurses' Station**.
• Click on **Patient List**.
• Click on **Get Report** next to Harry George's name.

11. Read the report. Is there anything else you wish the nurse would have included in the report regarding osteomyelitis? If so, what?

→ • Click on **Return to Nurses' Station**.
  • Click on **Medication Room**.
  • Click on **IV Storage**.
  • Click on the **Small Volume** bin and choose the IV antibiotic that is due to be given at 0800.

12. What dilution of this IV antibiotic is available for you to administer?

13. Over what amount of time should you infuse the IV antibiotic? (*Hint:* You may refer to the Drug Guide for this information.)

14. If you are using an IV pump to deliver this medication piggyback, what rate (mL per hour) will you select to give this infusion?

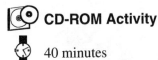 **CD-ROM Activity**

40 minutes

Exercise 2

  • Sign in to work at Pacific View Regional Hospital for Period of Care 2. (*Note:* If you are already in the virtual hospital from a previous exercise, click on **Leave the Floor** and then **Restart the Program** to get to the sign-in window.)
  • From the Patient List, select Harry George (Room 401).
  • Click on **Go to Nurses' Station**.
  • Click on **401**; inside Harry George's room, click on **Take Vital Signs**.

1. Below, record the vital sign findings you obtained.

B/P	SpO$_2$	Temp	HR	RR	Pain

→ • Click on **Patient Care** and then **Physical Assessment**.
  • Click on **Lower Extremities**.

    2. Complete a focused neurovascular assessment related to osteomyelitis and document your findings below.

 • Click on **Patient Care** and then **Nurse-Client Interactions**.

• Select and view the video titled **1120: Wound Management**. (*Note:* Check the virtual clock to see whether enough time has elapsed. You can use the fast-forward feature to advance the time by 2-minute intervals if the video is not yet available. Then click again on **Patient Care** and **Nurse-Client Interactions** to refresh the screen.)

    3. How does the nurse describe the progress of Harry George's wound condition? How does he respond?

    4. Based on your findings from questions 1 through 3, identify three priority nursing diagnoses for Harry George.

• Click on **Medication Room**.

• Click on **MAR** to determine what medications you need to administer to Harry George during this time period (1115-1200).

• Click on **Return to Medication Room**.

• Select the **IV Storage** icon.

• Click on the **Small Volume** bin and choose the IV antibiotic that is due to be given at 1200.

• Click **Put Medication in Tray** and then on **Close Bin**.

• Click on **View Medication Room**.

• Click on the **Drug** icon in the lower left corner of the screen.

5. Look up gentamicin in the Drug Guide. What must you assess before administering this drug? (*Hint:* Read the alert under Administration and Handling.)

→ • Click on **Return to Medication Room**.
  • Click on **Nurses' Station**.
  • Click on **Chart** and then on **401** for Harry George's chart.
  • Select the **Laboratory Reports** tab.

6. What are Harry George's most recent peak and trough levels?

7. Based on these results, what should your nursing actions be?

8. For what toxic side effects must you monitor?

9. What types of follow-up diagnostic tests should be anticipated for Harry George to determine how well the osteomyelitis is responding to therapy? What changes will occur in these diagnostic test results if therapy is effective?

10. If Harry George's infection does not respond to the antibiotic therapy, what other interventions would most likely be planned? Explain how these would benefit him.

11. Based on what you know and have read, what do you expect will be included in Harry George's discharge instructions and follow-up care to manage his osteomyelitis?

12. Based on Harry George's current living conditions, how do you think his care might best be managed?

LESSON **22** ——————————————

Intestinal Obstruction/ Colorectal Cancer

————————————————————

👓 **Reading Assignment:** Interventions for Clients with Noninflammatory Intestinal Disorders (Chapter 60)

Patient: Piya Jordan, Room 403

Goal: Utilize the nursing process to competently care for patients with noninflammatory intestinal disorders.

Objectives:

1. Correlate a patient's history and clinical manifestations with a diagnosis of intestinal obstruction.
2. Evaluate laboratory and diagnostic test results of a patient admitted with a noninflammatory intestinal disorder.
3. Plan appropriate nursing interventions for a patient with a nasogastric tube.
4. Prioritize nursing care for a patient with an intestinal obstruction.
5. Provide appropriate psychosocial interventions for a patient and family diagnosed with colon cancer.
6. Formulate an appropriate patient education plan for a postoperative patient with colorectal cancer.

In this lesson you will learn the essentials of caring for a patient admitted with an intestinal obstruction and diagnosed with colorectal cancer. You will explore the patient's history, evaluate presenting symptoms and treatment, plan appropriate nursing interventions, and develop an individualized teaching plan. Piya Jordan is a 68-year-old female admitted with nausea and vomiting for several days following weeks of poor appetite and increasing weakness.

✏️ **Clinical Preparation: Writing Activity**

⌚ 20 minutes

1. Describe the pathophysiology of fluid and electrolyte imbalances associated with an intestinal obstruction.

2. Compare and contrast a mechanical and nonmechanical intestinal obstruction.

    a. Mechanical obstruction

    b. Nonmechanical obstruction

3. How does the removal of polyps help to prevent colorectal cancer? (*Hint:* Describe the relationship between polyps and cancer development.)

4. Identify the most likely sites of metastasis for colorectal cancer.

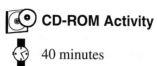 **CD-ROM Activity**

40 minutes

Exercise 1

- Sign in to work at Pacific View Regional Hospital for Period of Care 1. (*Note:* If you are already in the virtual hospital from a previous exercise, click on **Leave the Floor** and then **Restart the Program** to get to the sign-in window.)
- From the Patient List, select Piya Jordan (Room 403).
- Click on **Go to Nurses' Station**.
- Click on **Chart** and then on **403**.
- Click on **Emergency Department**.

1. What were Piya Jordan's presenting symptoms?

→ • Click on **History and Physical**.

2. What history of symptoms is recorded?

→ • Click on **Laboratory Reports**.

3. Document Piya Jordan's admission electrolyte results below and on the next page. Evaluate whether each of the results is normal, decreased, or increased. Offer your rationale for any abnormalities in the last column.

	Monday 2200	Decreased, Normal, or Increased?	Rationales for Abnormality
Sodium			
Potassium			
Chloride			
CO_2			

	Monday 2200	Decreased, Normal, or Increased?	Rationales for Abnormality
Creatinine			
BUN			
Amylase			

→ • Click on **Diagnostic Reports**.

4. What was the result of Piya Jordan's KUB? What do her air-fluid levels indicate?

5. Why was a CT scan of the abdomen ordered? What was the result?

6. What part of the bowel is the terminal ileum?

7. Was Piya Jordan's obstruction mechanical or nonmechanical? Explain.

8. If Piya Jordan had sought medical attention before the obstruction worsened, what other diagnostic testing might she have undergone? Explain what that test would show.

→ • Click on **History and Physical**.

9. Now that you know Piya Jordan has a colonic mass, let's look at her presenting symptoms again. Common clinical manifestations of colorectal cancer are listed below. Circle any that are consistent with her history or her physical examination findings on admission.

Incomplete evacuation	Anemia
Blood in stool	Fatigue
Narrowing of stools	Palpable mass
Change in stool	Pain
Straining to pass stools	Abdominal distention

→ • Click on **Physician's Orders**.

10. What IV fluid did the Emergency Department physician initially order? Why? (*Hint:* Review her vital signs in the ED documentation and relate these to fluid/electrolyte changes noted with intestinal obstruction.)

11. What else did the Emergency Department physician order to treat the intestinal obstruction? Explain the purpose of this intervention.

→ • Click on **Return to Nurses' Station**.
 • Click on **403** to enter Piya Jordan's room.
 • Click on **Patient Care** and then **Physical Assessment**.

12. Perform a focused abdominal assessment. Document your findings below.

13. Describe any additional assessments and/or interventions related to the NGT that you might do for Piya Jordan.

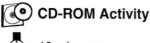 **CD-ROM Activity**

🕙 45 minutes

Exercise 2

• Sign in to work at Pacific View Regional Hospital for Period of Care 3. (*Note:* If you are already in the virtual hospital from a previous exercise, click on **Leave the Floor** and then **Restart the Program** to get to the sign-in window.)
• From the Patient List, select Piya Jordan (Room 403).
• Click on **Go to Nurses' Station**.
• Click on **Chart** and then on **403**.
• Click on **History and Physical**.

1. Below is a list of risk factors for colorectal cancer. Circle those that are documented in Piya Jordan's record.

    History of polyps   Age

    High-fat, low-fiber diet   Family history

    Inflammatory bowel disease

➡ • Click on **Laboratory Reports**.

2. Below, record Piya Jordan's admission H&H and interpret the results.

	Monday 2200	Decreased, WNL, or Increased?	Rationale for Abnormality
Hemoglobin			
Hematocrit			

➡ • Click on **Expired MARs**.

3. What was administered preoperatively to clean out Piya Jordan's bowel?

4. If her surgery had not been an emergency, describe the type of bowel prep you might have expected to administer. Why is this done?

➡ • Click on **Surgical Reports**.

5. Look at the operative report. Name and describe the surgical procedure.

6. If the tumor had been larger, what further surgery might Piya Jordan have needed? (*Hint:* See Table 60-2 in your textbook.)

7. What is the most likely cell type for Piya Jordan's cancer?

8. How will the physician know what kind of cancer the tumor is?

9. How would you classify Piya Jordan's tumor according to the Dukes' classification system? Explain.

 • Click on **Laboratory Results**.

10. Why did the physician order an amylase, lipase, and LFTs? What do the results demonstrate?

➤ • Click on **Return to Nurses' Station**.
• Click on **403** to enter Piya Jordan's room.
• Click on **Patient Care** and then **Nurse-Client Interactions**.
• Click on and view the video titled **1500: Preventing Complications**. (*Note:* Check the virtual clock to see whether enough time has elapsed. You can use the fast-forward feature to advance the time by 2-minute intervals if the video is not yet available. Then click again on **Patient Care** and **Nurse-Client Interactions** to refresh the screen.)

11. What nursing interventions are discussed during this brief video? Why are they appropriate for Piya Jordan?

➤ • Now select on and view the video titled **1540: Discharge Planning**. (*Note:* Check the virtual clock to see whether enough time has elapsed. You can use the fast-forward feature to advance the time by 2-minute intervals if the video is not yet available. Then click again on **Patient Care** and **Nurse-Client Interactions** to refresh the screen.)

12. Piya Jordan's daughter seems to be overwhelmed by her mother's illness and needs. What psychosocial interventions could the nurse plan to help the client and her daughter?

13. What would you teach the daughter regarding health promotion and preventing colon cancer in herself?

14. Describe appropriate teaching points for Piya Jordan before her discharge.

Malnutrition/Obesity

Patients: Harry George, Room 401
Piya Jordan, Room 403
Jacquline Catanazaro, Room 402

Goal: Utilize the nursing process to competently care for patients with nutritional disorders.

Objectives:

1. Identify patients at risk for malnutrition.
2. Perform a nutritional screening assessment on assigned patients.
3. Evaluate laboratory findings in relation to a patient's nutritional status.
4. Plan appropriate dietary interventions for a patient with malnutrition.
5. Identify a patient's risk factors related to obesity.
6. Formulate an appropriate patient education plan for an overweight patient.

In this lesson you will learn the essentials of caring for patients with nutritional disorders. You will explore each patient's history, perform a nutritional screening assessment, evaluate findings, and plan appropriate nursing interventions, including each patient's educational needs. Harry George is a 54-year-old male with a 4-year history of type 2 diabetes admitted with infection and swelling of his left foot. Piya Jordan is a 68-year-old female admitted with nausea and vomiting for several days following weeks of poor appetite and increasing weakness. Jacquline Catanazaro is a 45-year-old female admitted with an acute exacerbation of asthma.

Clinical Preparation: Writing Activity

10 minutes

1. What are the basal energy needs of a healthy adult?

2. Identify the seven Dietary Guidelines for Americans developed by the U.S. Department of Agriculture and the U.S. Department of Health and Human Services in 1995.

3. Describe the Food Guide Pyramid, including the number of servings recommended for each food group.

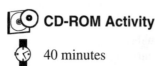 **CD-ROM Activity**

 40 minutes

Exercise 1

- Sign in to work at Pacific View Regional Hospital for Period of Care 1. (*Note:* If you are already in the virtual hospital from a previous exercise, click on **Leave the Floor** and then **Restart the Program** to get to the sign-in window.)
- From the Patient List, select Harry George (Room 401) and Piya Jordan (Room 403).
- Click on **Go to Nurses' Station**.
- Click on **Chart** and then on **401** for Harry George's record.
- Click on **History and Physical**.

1. What risk factors for malnutrition are noted in Harry George's H&P?

- Click on **Return to Nurses' Station**.
- Click on **Chart** and then on **403** for Piya Jordan's chart.
- Click on **History and Physical**.

2. What risk factors for malnutrition are noted in Piya Jordan's H&P?

 3. According to your textbook, a thorough assessment of a client's nutritional status should include what seven areas?

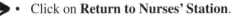

- Click on **Return to Nurses' Station**.
- Click on **401** to enter Harry George's room.
- Click on **Patient Care** and then **Physical Assessment**.

4. Although not every client needs a complete nutritional assessment, it is essential to identify clients at risk for nutritional problems through an initial nutritional screening. Perform a nutritional screening assessment on Harry George by answering the questions, noted as best practices in your textbook, in column 1 below and on the next two pages. Obtain as much information as possible by completing a physical assessment on this client and documenting your findings in column 2. Information that you are unable to currently assess for can be found by reading Harry George's History and Physical, the Nursing Admission form, and/or the EPR form. (*Note:* You will perform a similar assessment on Piya Jordan during Exercise 2 and record those findings in column 3.)

Screening Assessments	Harry George	Piya Jordan
General		
Does the client have any conditions that cause nutrient loss, such as malabsorption syndromes, draining abscesses, wounds, fistulas, or protracted diarrhea?		
Does the client have any conditions that increase the need for nutrients, such as fever, burn, injury, sepsis, or antineoplastic therapies?		
Has the client been on NPO status for 3 days or more?		
Is the client receiving a modified diet or a diet restricted in one or more nutrients?		

Screening Assessments	Harry George	Piya Jordan

Is the client being enterally or parenterally fed?

Does the client describe food allergies, lactose intolerance, or limited food preferences?

Has the client experienced a recent unexplained weight loss?

Is the client taking medications, either prescription, over-the-counter, or herbal/natural products?

Gastrointestinal

Does the client complain of nausea, indigestion, vomiting, diarrhea, or constipation?

Does the client exhibit glossitis, stomatitis, or esophagitis?

Does the client have difficulty chewing or swallowing?

Does the client have a partial or total gastrointestinal obstruction?

What is the client's state of dentition?

Cardiovascular

Does the client have ascites or edema?

Is the client able to perform activities of daily living?

Does the client have heart failure?

Does fluid input approximately equal fluid output? (*Hint:* Look at the EPR.)

Genitourinary

Does the client have an ostomy?

Is the client hemodialyzed or periotoneally dialyzed?

Screening Assessments	**Harry George**	**Piya Jordan**

Respiratory

Is the client receiving mechanical ventilatory support?

Is the client receiving oxygen via nasal prongs?

Does the client have chronic obstructive pulmonary disease (COPD) or asthma?

Integumentary

Does the client have nail or hair changes?

Does the client have rashes or dermatitis?

Does the client have dry or pale mucous membranes or decreased skin turgor?

Does the client have pressure areas on the sacrum, hips, or ankles?

Extremities

Does the client have pedal edema?

Does the client exhibit cachexia?

---

 5. Using Harry George's documented height and weight on admission, calculate his body mass index (BMI). (*Hint:* See page 1426 of your textbook.)

6. What is Harry George's albumin level?

7. Evaluate the results of your findings from questions 4, 5, and 6. Is Harry George malnourished or at risk for malnutrition? Explain how you came to your conclusion.

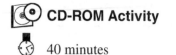 **CD-ROM Activity**

40 minutes

Exercise 2

- Sign in to work at Pacific View Regional Hospital for Period of Care 1. (*Note:* If you are already in the virtual hospital from a previous exercise, click on **Leave the Floor** and then **Restart the Program** to get to the sign-in window.)
- From the Patient List, select Harry George (Room 401) and Piya Jordan (Room 403).
- Click on **Go to Nurses' Station**.
- Click on **403** to enter Piya Jordan's room.
- Click on **Patient Care** and then **Physical Assessment**.

1. Now perform the same nutritional screening assessment on Piya Jordan as you did for Harry George earlier in this lesson. Obtain as much data as possible; then document your findings in the third column of the three-page table in Exercise 1, question 4. (*Remember:* Information that you are unable to currently assess for can be found by reading the History and Physical, the Nursing Admission form, and/or the EPR form.)

2. Calculate Piya Jordan's BMI based on her current height and weight.

3. What is her albumin level?

4. Evaluate the results of your findings from questions 1, 2, and 3. Is Piya Jordan malnourished or at risk for malnutrition? Explain how you came to your conclusion.

5. Compare and contrast your findings for Harry George and Piya Jordan. What are the similarities? What are the differences?

Similarities

Differences

6. What other laboratory tests would give you more information on Piya Jordan's and Harry George's nutritional status?

7. Identify two nursing diagnoses related to the malnourished status of these two clients.

8. What type of diet or dietary supplements would you recommend for these two clients?

 CD-ROM Activity

30 minutes

Exercise 3

- Sign in to work at Pacific View Regional Hospital for Period of Care 2. (*Note:* If you are already in the virtual hospital from a previous exercise, click on **Leave the Floor** and then **Restart the Program** to get to the sign-in window.)
- From the Patient List, select Jacquline Catanazaro (Room 402).
- Click on **Go to Nurses' Station**.
- Click on **Chart** and then on **402**.
- Click on **Nursing Admission**.

1. Record Jacquline Catanazaro's current height and weight below.

2. Calculate her BMI.

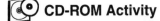 3. Is Jacquline Catanazaro's nutritional status normal, overweight, obese, or morbidly obese? (*Hint:* See page 1435 of the textbook.)

• Click on **History and Physical**.

4. What complication of obesity does Jacquline Catanazaro suffer from?

5. What other complications is she at risk for?

6. What are the contributing factors for her increased weight?

 • Click on **Return to Nurses' Station**.
 • Click on **MAR** and then on **402**.

7. Do any of the medications ordered for Jacquline Catanazaro cause weight gain? If so, explain below. (*Hint:* Return to the Nurses' Station and consult the Drug Guide.)

→ • Click on **Return to Nurses' Station**, then on **402** to enter Jacquline Catanazaro's room.
 • Click on **Patient Care** and then **Nurse-Client Interactions**.
 • Select and view the video titled **1140: Compliance—Medications**. (*Note:* Check the virtual clock to see whether enough time has elapsed. You can use the fast-forward feature to advance the time by 2-minute intervals if the video is not yet available. Then click again on **Patient Care** and **Nurse-Client Interactions** to refresh the screen.)

8. What concern does the client voice regarding her medications?

9. Evaluate the nurse's response. Was it appropriate? Was it accurate? Explain.

10. What else could the nurse have suggested to help this client lose weight?

11. If Jacquline Catanazaro was morbidly obese, what other treatment options might she have?

LESSON **24**

Diabetes Mellitus, Part 1

⟳ **Reading Assignment:** Interventions for Clients with Diabetes Mellitus (Chapter 68)

Patient: Harry George, Room 401

Goal: Utilize the nursing process to competently care for patients with diabetes mellitus.

Objectives:

1. Describe the pathophysiology of diabetes mellitus.
2. Compare and contrast the characteristics of type 1 and type 2 diabetes.
3. Identify the relationship between diabetes and other disease processes.
4. Evaluate a patient's risk factors for diabetes.
5. Assess a patient for short- and long-term complications of diabetes.
6. Develop an appropriate plan of care for a patient with type 2 diabetes.

In this lesson you will learn the essentials of caring for a patient admitted with complications related to diabetes mellitus. You will explore the patient's history, evaluate presenting symptoms and treatment, plan appropriate nursing interventions, and develop an individualized teaching plan. Harry George is a 54-year-old male with a 4-year history of type 2 diabetes admitted with infection and swelling of his left foot.

✎ **Clinical Preparation: Writing Activity**

⌚ 20 minutes

1. Describe the pathophysiology of diabetes mellitus and the basis for the resulting abnormalities in carbohydrate, protein, and fat metabolism.

2. Briefly define and summarize the etiologic differences between type 1 and type 2 diabetes mellitus.

Type 1 diabetes mellitus

Type 2 diabetes mellitus

3. Compare and contrast the distinguishing features of type 1 and type 2 diabetes mellitus (DM) by completing the table below.

Features	Type 1 DM	Type 2 DM
Insulin status		
Age		
Clinical presentation		
Antigen patterns		
Antibodies		
Treatment		
Body weight		
Former names		

CD-ROM Activity

45 minutes

Exercise 1

- Sign in to work at Pacific View Regional Hospital for Period of Care 1. (*Note:* If you are already in the virtual hospital from a previous exercise, click on **Leave the Floor** and then **Restart the Program** to get to the sign-in window.)
- From the Patient List, select Harry George (Room 401).
- Click on **Go to Nurses' Station**.
- Click on **Chart** and then on **401** for the correct chart.
- Click on **History and Physical**.

1. What risk factors for diabetes are noted in Harry George's history?

2. Describe the history of his present illness.

3. What is the relationship between the infection in Harry George's foot and his diabetes mellitus? (*Hint:* Read about chronic complications in textbook.)

- Click on **Laboratory Reports**.

4. What was Harry George's admitting blood sugar?

5. What abnormalities in his urinalysis results can be attributed to diabetes? Explain the relationship.

• Click on **Emergency Department**.

6. What factor in Harry George's recent history most likely contributed to his hyperglycemia? (*Hint:* Read the ED physician's notes for 1345.)

• Click on **Nursing Admission**.

7. Listed below are clinical manifestations of diabetes mellitus identified in the textbook. In column 2, indicate (with Yes or No) whether each manifestation is usually present in type 2 diabetes. Then indicate (with Yes or No) whether Harry George displays each manifestation based on the nurse's initial assessment.

Clinical Manifestations	Present in Type 2 DM? (Yes or No)	Experienced by Harry George? (Yes or No)
Polyuria		
Polydypsia		
Polyphagia		
Visual blurring		
Fatigue		
Weight loss		
Chronic complications		

8. To what extent does Harry George fit the typical picture of a client with type 2 diabetes mellitus?

• Click on **Return to Nurses' Station**.
• Click on **401** to enter Harry George's room.
• Click on **Patient Care** and then **Nurse-Client Interactions**.
• Select and view the video titled **0755: Disease Management**. (*Note:* Check the virtual clock to see whether enough time has elapsed. You can use the fast-forward feature to advance the time by 2-minute intervals if the video is not yet available. Then click again on **Patient Care** and **Nurse-Client Interactions** to refresh the screen.)

9. What does Harry George tell the nurse about his appetite?

10. What diet has been ordered for this client? (*Hint:* Review his chart.)

11. Describe the principles of this diet.

12. How might the client's alcohol intake affect his blood glucose levels?

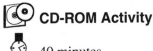

CD-ROM Activity

40 minutes

Exercise 2

- Sign in to work at Pacific View Regional Hospital for Period of Care 2. (*Note:* If you are already in the virtual hospital from a previous exercise, click on **Leave the Floor** and then **Restart the Program** to get to the sign-in window.)
- From the Patient List, select Harry George (Room 401).
- Click on **Go to Nurses' Station**.
- Click on **Chart** and then on **401**.
- Click on **Physician's Orders**.

1. What test is ordered that can be used to determine Harry George's control of diabetes mellitus? Describe the purpose of this test. How often should it be done?

2. What were the results of this test for Harry George? Based on these results, evaluate and explain how well his diabetes is controlled.

3. What implication does Harry George's level of glycemic control have for his future?

 • Click on **Return to Nurses' Station**.
• Click on **401** to enter Harry George's room.
• Click on **Patient Care** and then **Physical Assessment**.

4. Perform a head-to-toe assessment on Harry George. Document any abnormal results below.

Assessment Area	Assessment Results
Head & Neck	
Chest	
Back & Spine	
Upper Extremities	
Abdomen	
Pelvic	
Lower Extremities	

➜ • Click on **EPR** and **Login**. Choose **401** from the Patient drop-down menu and select **Neurologic** as the category.

5. Below, document any abnormal information obtained from the neurological assessment completed on Monday at 1835.

6. Describe the following potential long-term complications for diabetes mellitus.

Cardiovascular disease

Cerebrovascular disease

Peripheral vascular disease

Retinopathy

Neuropathy

Nephropathy

Erectile dysfunction

7. Does Harry George exhibit signs or symptoms that would alert you to the possibility of any of the long-term complications noted in question 6? If so, explain. (*Hint:* Consider your answers to questions 4 and 5 of this exercise, as well as question 5 in Exercise 1.)

 8. What patient teaching would you plan to offer Harry George for prevention of injury secondary to reduced sensation in his left foot? (*Hint:* See Chart 68-8 in the textbook.)

Diabetes Mellitus, Part 2

✍ **Reading Assignment:** Interventions for Clients with Diabetes Mellitus (Chapter 68)

Patient: Harry George, Room 401

Goal: Utilize the nursing process to competently administer medications prescribed to treat patients with diabetes mellitus.

Objectives:

1. Describe the pharmacologic therapy used for a patient with diabetes.
2. Evaluate a patient's response to insulin therapy.
3. Assess a patient for side effects of insulin therapy.
4. Describe the clinical manifestations of hypoglycemia as a side effect of insulin therapy.
5. Develop an individualized teaching plan for a patient with type 2 diabetes.

In this lesson you will learn the essentials regarding pharmacologic therapy for a patient admitted with complications related to diabetes mellitus. You will identify, describe, administer, and evaluate effects of prescribed antidiabetic medications. Harry George is a 54-year-old male with a 4-year history of type 2 diabetes. He was admitted with infection and swelling of his left foot.

Clinical Preparation: Writing Activity

🕐 30 minutes

1. For each of the various types of insulin listed below and on the next page, identify brand name, onset, peak, and duration.

Insulin Classification/ Generic Name	Brand Name	Onset (hour)	Peak (hour)	Duration (hour)
Rapid-Acting				
Insulin aspart				
Insulin lispro				
Insulin glulisine				

Insulin Classification/ Generic Name	Brand Name	Onset (hour)	Peak (hour)	Duration (hour)
Short-Acting				
Regular insulin				
Buffered regular insulin				
Intermediate-Acting				
Human insulin isophane				
Human insulin zinc				
Long-Acting				
Human insulin extended zinc				
Insulin glargine				

2. Below, identify the five classifications of oral hypoglycemic agents, as well as specific medications and mechanism of action for each classification.

Classification	Medications	Mechanism of Action

CD-ROM Activity

40 minutes

Exercise 1

- Sign in to work at Pacific View Regional Hospital for Period of Care 1. (*Note:* If you are already in the virtual hospital from a previous exercise, click on **Leave the Floor** and then **Restart the Program** to get to the sign-in window.)
- From the Patient List, select Harry George (Room 401).
- Click on **Go to Nurses' Station**.
- Click on **Chart** and then on **401**.
- Click on **Emergency Department**.

1. What medication was ordered to control Harry George's diabetes?

2. How would you give the IV insulin? (*Hint:* You can access the Drug Guide by clicking on the **Drug** icon in the lower left corner of the screen in the Nurses' Station.)

3. Find the ED physician progress notes for Monday at 1345. What does the physician plan to order for the sliding scale insulin coverage?

➡ • Click on **Physician's Orders**.

4. Look at these orders for Monday at 1345. What was the actual sliding scale insulin order?

➡ • Click on **Return to Nurses' Station**.
- Click on **Kardex** and then on **401** to access the correct record.

5. According to the Kardex, how often should the capillary blood glucose be tested?

- Click on **Return to Nurses' Station**.
- Click on **MAR** and then on **401** for Harry George's records.

6. According to the MAR, when should the insulin sliding scale be administered? What was the time of this order?

7. What would you do regarding the inconsistencies identified above?

8. What problems might you anticipate for Harry George if he does not receive insulin coverage at bedtime?

- Click on **Return to Nurses' Station**.
- Click on **401** to enter Harry George's room.
- Click on **Clinical Alerts**.

9. What is the clinical alert for 0730?

Prepare and administer the sliding scale insulin for this glucose level by following these steps:

• Click **Medication Room** on the bottom of the screen.
• Click **MAR** or **Review MAR** at any time to verify how much insulin to administer based on sliding scale. (*Hint:* Remember to look at the patient name on the MAR to make sure you have the correct patient's records—you must click on correct room number within the MAR.) Click on **Return to Medication Room** after reviewing the correct MAR.
• Click on **Unit Dosage** and then on drawer **401** for Harry George's medications.
• Select **Insulin Regular**, put medication on tray, and then close the drawer.
• Click **View Medication Room**.
• Click on **Preparation** and choose the correct medication to administer. Click **Prepare**.
• Click **Next**, choose the correct patient to administer this medication to, and click **Finish**.
• You can click on **Review Your Medications** and then on **Return to Medication Room** when ready. Once you are back in the Medication Room, you may go directly to Harry George's room by clicking on **401** at the bottom of the screen.
• Click on **Patient Care**.
• Click on **Medication Administration** and follow the steps in the Administration Wizard to complete the insulin administration.

10. How much insulin should be administered?

11. What is the preferred site of administration for fastest absorption?

12. Fill in the table below regarding the insulin you just administered.

	Expected Length of Time	Actual Time After 0730 Dose
Onset		
Peak		
Duration		

13. At what time would Harry George be at most risk for hypoglycemia? Describe the clinical manifestations that would indicate this acute complication.

14. While you are preparing to administer Harry George's insulin, he asks you why he is taking this since he did not use insulin at home. How would you answer this?

15. For what side effects should you monitor Harry George related to his insulin regimen?

 CD-ROM Activity

40 minutes

Exercise 2

- Sign in to work at Pacific View Regional Hospital for Period of Care 4. (*Note:* If you are already in the virtual hospital from a previous exercise, click on **Leave the Floor** and then **Restart the Program** to get to the sign-in window.)
- Click on **Chart** and then on **401** for Harry George's chart. (*Remember:* You are not able to visit patients or administer medications during Period of Care 4. You are able to review patients' records only.)
- Click on **Nurse's Notes**.

1. Read the notes for Wednesday at 1730. What does the client request regarding glyburide?

2. How would you respond to the client's demands?

3. How often did Harry George take the glyburide at home?

4. Why do you think this was increased in the hospital? What concerns might you have regarding this increase? (*Hint:* This client is also receiving insulin.)

5. What classification of oral hypoglycemics does glyburide belong to?

6. For what side effects of glyburide should you assess Harry George? (*Hint:* For help, click on the **Drug Guide** located on the counter in the Nurses' Station.)

7. What specific patient teaching points should you give this client regarding glyburide?

→ • Click on **Laboratory Reports**.

8. Below, document Harry George's blood glucose and insulin administration since admission to the medical-surgical unit. (*Hint:* You may have to review the expired MARs in the chart to verify whether insulin was given for HS glucose measurement on Tuesday.)

Date/Time	Blood Glucose Level	Amount of Regular Insulin Administered

9. Based on Harry George's pattern of blood glucose levels, would you evaluate his current therapy as effective? If not, how might the physician further treat his diabetes?

10. If you were reviewing the chart orders and the EPR on Wednesday evening and found the information recorded in the table in question 8, what would you be ethically and legally bound to report?

Notes:

Notes:

Notes: